Wal

London's

Medical History

Walking London's
Medical History

Second edition

Nick Black

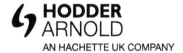

HODDER
ARNOLD
AN HACHETTE UK COMPANY

First published in Great Britain in 2006 by Royal Society of Medicine Press Ltd
This second edition published in 2012 by
Hodder Arnold, an imprint of Hodder Education, a division of Hachette UK

338 Euston Road, London NW1 3BH

http://www.hodderarnold.com

British Library Cataloguing in Publication Data
A catalogue record for this book is available from the British Library

Library of Congress Cataloging-in-Publication Data
A catalog record for this book is available from the Library of Congress

ISBN-13   978-1-4441-7243-0
1 2 3 4 5 6 7 8 9 10

Commissioning Editor:	Joanna Koster
Project Editor:	Stephen Clausard
Production Controller:	Joanna Walker
Cover Design:	Amina Dudhia
Indexer:	Lisa Footitt

Back cover image © Jeffrey Blackler/Alamy

Typeset in Adobe Caslon Roman 9 pts by Datapage (India) Pvt. Ltd.
Printed and bound in India

What do you think about this book? Or any other Hodder Arnold title?
Please visit our website: www.hodderarnold.com

For Pippa

About the author

Nick Black is Professor of Health Services Research at the London School of Hygiene & Tropical Medicine (University of London). He is one of the leading academics in the UK on health services, having published several books and over 200 articles in medical journals. He is the founding co-editor of the *Journal of Health Services Research & Policy*, a leading international journal, and edited a series of 20 books on Understanding Public Health. He advises the Department of Health on quality assessment and chairs the National Advisory Group for Clinical Audit & Enquiries. Apart from health care policy, his interests include history, architecture, cooking and Arsenal. He is married and lives in north London.

Contents

Acknowledgements

I am most grateful for the help and advice I received from: Terence Spurr and Riccard Parsonson (London Ambulance Service Museum); Claire Torkington (Camden Primary Care Trust); Fiona Bourne (Royal College of Nursing); Rachel Bairsto (British Dental Association Museum); Stephanie McNamara (General Medical Council); Susan Scott (Royal College of Paediatrics & Child Health); Philip Walker (Medical Protection Society); Adam Hall (Clerkenwell Medical Mission); Andrea Peace (Chartered Society of Physiotherapy); Victoria North (Royal Free Hospital Archives Centre); Nicholas Baldwin (Great Ormond Street Hospital Museum); Peter Morrell (Stoke on Trent College); Steve Wilson (National Hospital for Neurology & Neurosciences); Syeda Begum (Portland Hospital); Marvin Sturridge (Middlesex Hospital); Louise Boden, David Starke and Annie Lindsay (University College London Hospitals Trust); Richard Bowden (Howard de Walden Management Ltd); Wendy Butler and Gill Furlong (University College London); Pardip Kaur (World Electro Homeopathic Association); Clive Coward (Wellcome Trust Library); Adrian Autton (Westminster Archives Centre); Susan Isaac (King's College London); Joy Sharman (St Martin's Hospital, Canterbury); Ian Isherwood, Ed McKie, Chris Marshall (Eastry), Julie Deller (Deal), John Rogers (Deal), David Collyer (Deal), Dawn Crouch (Westgate), Harold Gough (Herne Bay Historical Records Society), Henrietta Curtis and Caroline Royds. Thanks also to Joanna Koster and Stephen Clausard at Hodder Arnold, and to Carrie Walker.

Foreword

London was once known as a vast hospital, in which its patients (or inhabitants) were never wholly well. The city was in essence a harmful and dirty place, a site for contagion and for epidemic distempers. It was a victim of fever in every sense. In this colourful and scholarly account, Nick Black examines the highways and bye-ways of London's medical past and he invites you to walk upon the haunted ground in search of the more surprising and gruesome episodes in the city's long history. The stories told along the route of this pilgrimage are of intense interest, reflecting as they do the continual battle against sickness and disease that engaged generation after generation of Londoners. The city is now a much more sturdy and healthy place, as the author makes clear, but anyone interested in its unwholesome and insalubrious past will wish to read this book. It is an anatomy upon the historical body of London.

Peter Ackroyd

Permissions

Historical Publications Ltd for figures on pages 6, 54, 198, 206 and 217.

Peter Higginbotham (www.workhouses.org.uk) for figures on pages 11, 236 and 253.

King's College School of Medicine Library Services for figure on page 20.

Wellcome Trust Medical Photographic Library for figures on pages 23, 32, 43, 52, 56, 60, 67, 73, 81, 92, 99, 118, 149, 199 and 222.

Islington Local History Centre for figures on pages 51 and 209.

The Trustees of Wesley's Chapel, City Road, London for figure on page 58.

Museum & Archive Service, Great Ormond Street Hospital for Children NHS Trust for figure on page 83.

City of Westminster Archives Centre for figure on page 108.

Hunterian Museum, Royal College of Surgeons of England for figure on page 124.

University College Hospitals NHS Foundation Trust Archives for figure on page 136.

The Estate of Abram Games for figure on page 203.

Museum of the Royal Pharmaceutical Society of Great Britain for figure on page 215.

London Metropolitan Archives for figures on pages 70, 111 and 146.

The history of health care

Introduction

The history of health care is complex, confusing and contested. While the 'great men of medicine' have made and continue to make important contributions to shaping health services, we can only understand why we have the services we have by looking beyond the contributions made by doctors. Many others have also had an influence: architects, politicians, ambulance staff, pharmacists, midwives, clerics, nurses, the monarchy, lawyers, philanthropists, writers … And health care is more than hospitals and dispensaries, infirmaries and health centres. It's also royal colleges, trades unions, medical schools, nurses' homes, coroners' courts, regulatory bodies, nursing sisterhoods, ambulance stations, patients' organisations, medical societies, medical missions, funding bodies, research institutes, nursing schools, examination halls … This book challenges the importance traditionally attached to some places and events, not to denigrate them but to put them in context and to recognise the importance of other, frequently neglected contributions. It also aims to entertain.

To enhance our understanding, we usually sit and read books or, nowadays, surf the internet. But it's more fun to go out and literally visit the past, see the buildings where events unfolded and transport yourself back in time. And for the history of health care in England,

there is nowhere better to do this than London. For it was in London that most of the key developments took place. It was here that the key battles were fought over health care policies, where conflicts were resolved and where many innovations occurred. Although some of the important buildings in the history of health care have been destroyed, many remain.

The book has three aims. First, through a series of seven walks in central London, it aims to tell the story of how health services developed from medieval times to the present day. Second, the walks aim to help preserve our legacy, as former health care buildings are increasingly converted into hotels, offices, homes and shops, with public knowledge of their original function in danger of being lost. And third, it aims to increase understanding of the current challenges we face in trying to improve health care in the 21st century. There are more lessons to be learnt from the past than has traditionally been accepted.

Ten general observations

As you explore London, discovering the history of its health services, several common characteristics should become clear. Some you may already be aware of; others may come as a surprise. There are ten features of health care that transcend particular historical periods and specific areas of London, and act as a guide to making sense of what is a complex story.

Health care is everywhere. The more you explore, the more you find. In some parts of London, almost every street has witnessed some activity involving the provision or the funding or the management of health care. This links to the second observation, that throughout history *large numbers of people have been engaged in health care*, depending on it for a livelihood. Add in all those who care for relatives and friends, and there are few of us who are not at some time involved in some capacity.

Despite the longevity of some of the best-loved institutions, *health care facilities are far from static and fixed*. They grow, merge, divide and move around the city driven by shifts in population and other social trends. As London broke out from the confines of the city walls in the 17th century, health services were carried along on this centrifugal wave. As the aristocracy and emerging mercantile class moved west from the city in the 19th century, so the epicentre of medical London pursued them, first to Holborn and Bloomsbury, then on to Marylebone.

While the British have made notable contributions to the evolution of health care worldwide, *the origin of many key developments in British health care lies overseas*: the way care is funded (voluntary hospitals originated in France); the way professionals learn (medical societies came from Italy; anatomical dissection from France; postgraduate education from Vienna); the

way care is managed (nursing sisterhoods derive from Germany); new technologies (forceps – and as a result, the creation of obstetrics – came from France; smallpox inoculation from Turkey); and the way care is organised (hospitals for children were introduced from France, Germany and Turkey). Health care has always been an international activity.

Health care is and always has been an industry. Despite many practitioners pursuing a vocation, some driven by religious devotion, health services have always attracted entrepreneurs who have seen the opportunities for a lucrative business, given the often desperate state of the potential customers. From the less scrupulous clerics running medieval hospitals, through the masters of private madhouses and the proprietors of private theatres of anatomy in the 18th century, to modern-day pharmaceutical companies and hospital corporations, there have always been those who have sought and succeeded in making money out of health care.

Related to this, *health care providers compete with one another for income and status*, be it competition between hospitals, or between hospitals and primary care. Although hospitals and their staff are reluctant to be seen by the public to be competing, there has always been a 'healthy rivalry' as institutions compete to employ the most eminent, accomplished staff and attract the most income. For example, in the 1830s, Charing Cross Hospital refused to help King's

College Medical School because it already had plans to set up its own medical school in competition. With competition for limited funds, some hostility is inevitable.

The distinction between licensed and unlicensed practitioners is not as clear and fixed as the former believe or wish. While doctors, nurses and other licensed professions have always seen a clear distinction between themselves and unlicensed 'quacks, mountebanks and charletans', the latter have made important contributions to the development of formal health care, including the establishment of ophthalmology and of the first Ear, Nose & Throat hospital, as well as the introduction of electrotherapy and hydrotherapy. In addition, lay people (often in the face of professional opposition) have led some key innovations such as establishing the first hospital for those paralysed or suffering from epilepsy, the introduction of family planning, and the provision of physiotherapy in the community. More recently, lay or patients' organisations have pioneered hospices and palliative care.

Although a series of walks inevitably limits the perspective to the confines of the city, it is essential to recognise that *no city is an island.* Throughout history, cities have depended on their rural hinterland in two principal ways. The countryside has provided a healthy retreat, be it the tea gardens and 'medicinal' spas of the 17th century, sea-bathing facilities in

the 18th and 19th centuries, or TB sanatoria and convalescent homes in the 20th century. It has also provided somewhere for confining those excluded from the city because they were deemed to threaten the health and safety of others – those who were mentally ill (or incapacitated) or infectious. The great 19th century asylums and infectious disease hospitals that ringed the city are lasting monuments to such health care policies. The motoring tour of Kent introduces you not only to these facilities, but also to how the health care needs of those living outside London and the needs of the military were met.

Most of the challenges that health services face have persisted for centuries. Most contemporary issues would have been familiar to our forbears:

- *governance or control of institutions*
  Struggles over who manages hospitals are nothing new, although nowadays this rarely results in walkouts by doctors or mass sackings by managers. In medieval hospitals, conflict between the Church and the Crown even led to armed takeovers. In the 19th century, disputes in voluntary hospitals between lay governors and doctors arose over who selected the patients. Conflict also arose when nursing was contracted out by lay governors to religious sisterhoods because many of the doctors resented the power and control the nurses were

granted, despite the obvious improvements the nurses produced.

- *insufficient funds*
Funds have never been sufficient, reflecting the fact that the demand for health care has exceeded and always will exceed the supply of funds. All that has changed over time is the mix of methods used to raise funds, which in turn reflects changes in attitudes towards social equity. In every age, people have searched for new sources of funds, but the only option is to adjust and readjust the mix of patient payments, private insurance, social insurance, taxation and donations.

- *interprofessional rivalry*
Disputes over who each profession can treat, what treatments they can employ, and what activities each profession can charge for have been going on for centuries. Some rivalries have been resolved, such as those between physicians, surgeons and apothecaries, whereas others persist, such as those between doctors and nurses, between obstetricians and midwives, and between allopathic (biomedical) and alternative practitioners.

And finally, *health services have been influenced by many external factors.* These influences extend from social attitudes to the role of women to religious beliefs, from developments in transport to wartime bombing, and from immigration to beliefs about the cause of disease. And at times it has been a two-way process: the professionalisation of nursing contributed to wider societal changes in women's role and status; and dependence on immigrant health care workers has affected public attitudes to immigration and race.

Drivers of change

Although the challenges that health care faces have altered little over time, there have been profound and at times dramatic changes in the way services are funded, governed, structured, located and organised. There have even been changes in what is considered health care. To make sense of the places you visit and the accounts of past events, it helps to be aware of what the principal drivers of change have been and, for the most part, continue to be.

Changing conceptions of illness and its causes

The way we have conceived the nature and cause of disease has profoundly affected health care. Galen's view, which held sway until the 19th century, considered that disease resulted from an imbalance of the four humours (key fluids) – blood, choler (yellow bile), phlegm and black bile – which could be corrected by bleeding, purging and herbal remedies, activities that did not necessitate the construction of hospitals or specialised buildings. Alongside these, belief in the therapeutic benefits of fresh air and sea-water led to the development of medicinal spas, sea-bathing establishments, convalescent homes and sanatoria. While these interventions have little part to play in modern biomedicine, such beliefs underlie many contemporary 'alternative or complementary' health services.

The impact of medical beliefs on health services can also be seen in our changing views of infection, from belief in contagion, through that of miasma (foul air) to germ theory. Such shifts in belief led to changes in where hospitals for patients with infectious diseases were located and how they were designed. Similarly, as views of those who were mentally ill evolved, so have services for those afflicted: first viewed as dangerous, necessitating custodial confinement; then seen as treatable, needing protection in a safe, healing environment (asylum); next considered hopeless, so abandoned in 'warehouses' with minimal care; and now believed to have a manageable condition, hence 'care in the community' facilitated by technological development (new drugs).

Introduction of new technologies

As health care technology has developed, the requirements for housing it have altered. Up until the 19th century, most health care could be delivered in domestic settings. Affluent patients were treated in their own homes. Others were treated in dispensaries and hospitals, most of which initially occupied domestic buildings adapted to the task. However, as new technologies were adopted, health services had to adapt. Purpose-built hospitals were constructed in the 19th century, driven by the concerns of sanitarians (who believed in miasma) who sought to minimise the risks of hospital-acquired infections. However, technology had only a limited impact: the National Temperance Hospital, built in 1881, used its boardroom, complete with an open fire, as the operating theatre. In contrast, since 1900, technological advances have been a major factor in shaping the development both of hospitals and of professions (e.g. radiographers as a profession were created to undertake X-ray investigations). And the current expansion of primary care is partly led by new technologies that allow traditional hospital care to be provided in the community.

Socio-demographic changes

The most profound demographic change in London has been the increase in size of the population as industrialisation drew impoverished people in from rural areas. Growth in the number of urban poor led to the development of ever-larger workhouses that, inevitably, included many who were sick and infirm. The early workhouse infirmaries provided little in the way of health care, but by the late 19th century huge, purpose-built infirmaries had been constructed, separate from the workhouses. Many such buildings survived into the 20th century, becoming public hospitals serving wider populations.

Another feature of the changing demography of London has been immigration. The authorities made no special provision for non-English-speaking residents (or visitors), so their needs were met through self-help initiatives. Several immigrant groups, from the Scots in the 1670s and French Huguenots in the 1710s to the Japanese in the 1980s, established dispensaries and hospitals for themselves, staffed by members of their own community. As groups have integrated, their need for separate provision has lessened or disappeared, as have the separate services.

Another example of the influence of socio-demographic changes was the growing number of single, working people in rented accommodation (who had migrated to London from the provinces) with no family to care for them when they fell ill. This encouraged the establishment of private nursing homes in the late 19th century.

Social attitudes

Many changes in health services have been driven by changes in social attitudes. In the 18th century, acceptance by the aristocracy and the *nouveaux riches* of their responsibility to those less fortunate was a major factor in the establishment and development of voluntary hospitals and dispensaries. In the 19th century, lack of apparent concern about high childhood death rates was challenged, leading to the provision of health care for children.

In the early 20th century, a commitment to eugenics (held by Marie Stopes and the British Medical Association, among others) lay behind the establishment of family-planning services. However, some deeply held beliefs could be sacrificed in acts of enlightened pragmatism: women's exclusion from medicine and ambulance work was temporarily suspended during World War I when men had gone to fight at the front.

Apart from the Church's direct involvement in providing health care (discussed below), religious attitudes also affected health services indirectly before 1900: services for women with venereal disease were as much about 'rescuing' women in need of redemption as about curing disease.

Religion

Clerics and churches have been involved in the provision of health care for centuries – from medieval hospitals, through small charitable hospitals in the 19th century to, in the 20th century, hospices. Health care has always sought to provide both spiritual salvation and physical care; what has varied is the balance between the two. For example, in the 18th century, clerics often provided some health care alongside their spiritual support (as they were often the only educated members of the local community). John Wesley, the founder of Methodism, ran a dispensary and even became a leading electrotherapist in Britain. In the late 19th century, churches established medical missions in London, to serve the poorest in society for whom there was no other provision, even if the help was inevitably limited to 'saving the souls of the dying'.

Religion has also been influential through the governance of health services: bishops retained the power to license surgeons up until 1713; parishes were responsible for administering the Poor Law until 1834; voluntary dispensaries and hospitals had clerics among their governors; and voluntary hospitals were partly dependent for income on the Hospital Sunday Fund, derived from church collections. But perhaps the most significant influence came from the religious nursing sisterhoods, which, in the second half of the 19th century, led the transformation of the voluntary hospitals into properly managed organisations.

Finance

Financial considerations have always influenced the location and organisation of health services. Many leading doctors moved their homes and practices from the City to Holborn in the early 19th century, and then on to Marylebone, to keep close to their wealthy, paying patients. Similarly, the voluntary general hospitals that were established in the first half of the 19th century sought locations where they could benefit from the new railway termini that brought patients into central London. Land prices have also had an influence. For example, when City Road was created in 1761, hospitals in the overcrowded City took advantage of the opportunity to expand by moving to the relatively cheap land

that became available near this new thoroughfare.

Pressure to make ends meet has meant that health care providers (such as hospitals) have been forced to be opportunistic and pragmatic. Despite the intention of voluntary hospitals to serve exclusively the working poor, the enticement of extra income by accepting more affluent patients who could be charged proved irresistible (a situation that has continued within the NHS). Meanwhile, since medieval times, the principal funders of health care have, not unreasonably, tried to influence the services they have paid for. In the late 19th century, funders such as the Hospital Saturday Fund and the King's Fund tried to shape voluntary hospitals by encouraging mergers, relocations and the introduction of stricter checks on patients' entitlements by the introduction of Lady Almoners. At the same time, from 1867, the Metropolitan Asylums Board successfully reorganised the services it funded – for infectious diseases and mental incapacity – in a move that was a precursor to full-blown strategic planning by the NHS from 1948.

Physical environment

Changes in the physical environment have played their part in shaping health services. The need to widen roads to accommodate increased traffic and the introduction of horse-drawn trams forced hospitals, such as the London Ophthalmic Hospital in Upper Moorfields, to move. Later the construction of the great railway termini meant that the London

Smallpox Hospital and the London Fever Hospital had to find new locations, and construction of the London Underground had a similar impact on the Great Northern Hospital. Meanwhile, attempts at slum clearance and improvements in road connections, such as the creation of City Road, provided opportunities for new sites for hospitals. One other factor to shape the physical environment occurred in the 1940s, namely aerial bombing during World War II. Many hospitals suffered serious damage that led to their demise, their relocation or major reconstruction. The bomb-sites that littered London also provided new opportunities for health services to be developed.

War

War and the military have had profound effects on civilian health services in several ways. Military hospitals have pioneered innovations in both design and organisation, perhaps because of the added incentive of the consequences of failing to maintain a competent fighting force. New ideas originated not only in the large military hospitals in Britain, but also in the field hospitals across the world, most notably from Nightingale's experiences in the Crimean War.

War has also affected health care in other ways. It has cut off supplies: the shortage of leeches from France during the Napoleonic wars necessitated a change of policy such that leeches had to be re-used rather than discarded after one use. War has resulted in the arrival and settlement

of refugees who have introduced different approaches to health care: the French Huguenots introduced the concept of voluntary support for services from affluent members of the community, for example. War has also highlighted previously neglected health problems: during World War I, the threat of venereal disease to the health of the fighting force so alarmed the government that specialist services were rapidly established. And war has raised people's expectations: the creation of the NHS was partly driven by the need to provide a 'home fit for heroes'.

Health care professions

The ambitions and aspirations of the health care professions, most notably doctors, have also helped shape health care. Persuading government to introduce licences to practise had the professions' desired effect of limiting the number of practitioners available, thus helping to protect their income and status. Self-determination of their own training requirements has had consequences for staffing levels in hospitals, for workload and responsibilities, and even for hospital architecture. For example, doctors who served voluntary hospitals in an honorary (unpaid) capacity enjoyed a considerable income from the fees paid to them by students who accompanied them on the wards. But the large number of students on teaching rounds meant that wards had to be designed to accommodate the large entourages, otherwise the hospital risked losing its 'star' doctors. Teaching needs have also meant that doctors have sometimes selected patients on the basis of their value as teaching material rather than their clinical need.

Professional demands for better employment conditions have, not surprisingly, had an impact on the finances and organisation of care. In the mid-19th century, governors of voluntary hospitals were ambivalent about the introduction of nursing sisterhoods: they recognised the necessity if the hospital was to improve the quality of its care, but resented the increased staffing levels the sisterhoods demanded (and got). Later on, in 1920, when the matron at Charing Cross Hospital negotiated a day off a week for nurses, all other hospitals had to follow suit despite the increased cost.

The walks

To help untangle the complexity of the history of health care, each walk described in this book has a major theme (as well as some minor ones), which is described in an introductory essay to the walk. Inevitably, the sequence of sites along the walks is largely determined by geography, making it impossible to create a chronological story. One aim of the introductory essays is therefore to provide an overview of the themes to enable you to see where a particular building or event fits in the chronology of events. The main themes of the walks are:

Walk 1: Church, Crown and City
    How these three powers have competed with one another to control health services and to influence health care policy.
Walk 2: The lost hospitals of St Luke's
    How the fortune of districts and of hospitals can change dramatically over time.
Walk 3: A cradle of reform
    How in a 40-year period health care was radically altered by the events that took place in one small area of London.
Walk 4: The challenging isle
    How individual creativity and entrepreneurship can shape the development of health care.
Walk 5: Merge or move
    How hospitals have faced the unavoidable choice between merger with larger neighbours or migration away from central London.
Walk 6: From trades to professions
    How health care trades transformed themselves into professions and defined their territories and rights.
Walk 7: 'Merrie Islington' to 'the contagion of numbers'
    How primary care developed from a market of unlicensed healers to a coordinated, multiprofessional system.

As far as possible, the walks concentrate on surviving buildings, minimising the number of past sites where nothing remains to be seen. Where past sites are included, an illustration of the lost building is usually provided. Little attention is paid to where some of the 'great men of medicine' used to live, whether or not their former homes sport a commemorative plaque. The aim is to give you a feel of how health services were intricately embedded in the physical and social fabric of London, and how extensive their presence has always been.

Dividing up central London into manageable walks was not a random exercise. They were determined by identifying the geographical boundaries of each theme. For example, the development of the professions was largely confined to the eastern half of Marylebone. This process suggests that connections between places and events are not due to chance but can partly be understood and explained by consideration of the physical, social and economic characteristics of an area.

All seven walks are presented in a similar format. Directions (together with a map) guide you from site to site. The text aims to provide you with sufficient information to appreciate the importance and contribution associated with the buildings you see. Additional background information on generic topics, such as voluntary general hospitals, providing a broad overview, is presented in boxes throughout the text. As all the walks are in central London, you will encounter numerous opportunities for refreshment, so no attempt has been made to suggest places where you may wish to take a break.

Before setting off, two warnings. First, these walks are about health care and not about public health. Therefore, little or no attention is paid to the many dramatic measures that have been taken to improve people's health through building river embankments, constructing sewage systems, providing clean water and reliable food supplies, and many other actions. And second, even seven walks cannot cover the whole of central London. You may be surprised that some major health care sites, such as St Bartholomew's Hospital or Apothecaries' Hall, do not appear. This simply reflects the choice of themes explored, and is not a rejection of the importance of such sites. However, it does reflect the over-riding ethos of the book, that of challenging the relative importance that traditional accounts have attached to some places and events. The book takes as much interest in one of the six ambulance stations built in 1915 by the London County Council as it does in the grandest teaching hospital.

And when you have walked the streets of London, you can complete the story of how the health care needs of Londoners have been met by spending three days in north and east Kent on a motoring tour. This will also enable you to see how health care was provided for those living outside the metropolis, how the needs of the army and navy have been met, and the extensive network of medieval hospitals that provided care for sick pilgrims who flocked to shrines with 'healing properties'.

[The author would be interested to hear your thoughts and comments at nick.black@lshtm.ac.uk]

Walk 1: Church, Crown and City

The history of this area embodies the key shifts of power from the Church to the Crown and then to the City. On this walk, you will see how the fortunes of these three forces have changed over time, how they have competed with one another despite their mutual dependency and the impact that this has had on the development and provision of health care.

Before 1200 the Church was the principal provider of institutional care, reflecting both its Christian mission and its immense power. There were over 100 churches in the city, and much of the land outside the city walls was owned by religious orders. Between 1100 and 1300, the bishops built themselves 45 ecclesiastical palaces, many along the river south of the Strand, to provide themselves with a London base for their political dealings. On a more altruistic note, the Church established hospitals outside the city walls. Apart from those with a general remit such as St Bartholomew's and St Thomas', ten were specifically for leprosy sufferers.

However, a key source of the Church's power was to prove its undoing. The concept of purgatory instilled fear in the affluent for it promised suffering for the rich and unrepentant, who in the after-life would be judged by the poor and the meek. This fear was exploited by the Church, which offered salvation (through the sale of indulgences) to those who bestowed gifts during their lives and endowments on their death. The rich would endow chantries, in essence paying the living to pray for their souls after death. And what better to endow than hospitals with their poor, infirm inmates with nothing better to occupy their time than praying.

The Church had to coexist with the Crown. The power of the latter fluctuated depending on the skill and ability of the monarch, the extent to

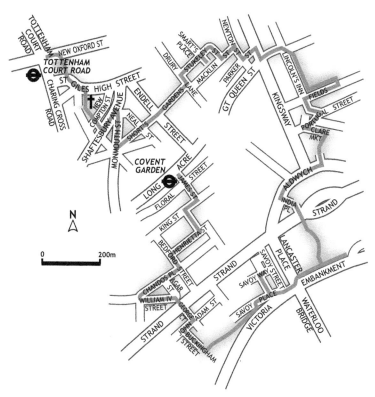

which the monarch was distracted by overseas exploits, and the level of control over their local agents – the sheriffs and sergeants. Although at times the Crown was in conflict with the Church, there was an underlying mutual dependence based on common interests. After all, monarchs were as susceptible to the threats of purgatory as others. And everyone lived in fear of pestilence and disease.

Throughout the 12th and 13th centuries, the power of the third major player, the City, was developing. As manufacturing and trade grew, guilds to protect and promote tradesmen's interests were established. These were voluntary organisations offering mutual support. By 1200 there were already 19, and this grew to over 100 by 1400 (including the Barbers' Company). Alongside these, self-governance of the City was achieved with the right to appoint their own sheriff (the Crown's representative) and to establish a commune with a mayor as leader. The mayor was both the voice of the City and the King's agent. The City's powers were confirmed in the Magna Carta in 1215.

Until 1500, the Church, Crown and City coexisted in an, at times, uneasy partnership. The Church continued to be the provider of hospitals for the sick and destitute. The only other health care was provided by a collection of self-taught healers including bone-setters, corn-cutters, herbalists, midwives, barbers and tooth-pullers. Although the power of the Church was increasingly viewed as exploitative, it was not until other circumstances (Henry VIII's desire for a divorce) arose in the 1530s that the Crown moved against the Church. The Reformation exploited widespread anti-clerical feelings, some of which arose from the Church's corrupt governance of hospitals. Alms (donations) intended for the poor and needy were seen to be supporting clerics and bishops.

Starting in 1534, the Crown systematically swept away religious establishments, including the ecclesiastical palaces that lined the Strand. These were handed over to noblemen supportive of the monarch. Also destroyed were the estimated 600 hospitals in England. Often the chapel was retained and became a parish church. In other instances, no trace remained. However, thanks to the intervention of the City, who found the sick and infirm literally on their doorsteps, five hospitals were refounded as secular, royal hospitals, most notably St Bartholomew's, St Thomas' and St Mary of Bethlehem. In an example of cooperation between Crown and City, the governance of the royal hospitals became the responsibility of the City. The dependence of the Crown on the City for finance was balanced by the City's need for endorsement of its right to self-govern. This ensured that tensions never extended to outright conflict. Their relationship has been likened to a bickering marriage in which each needed the other.

During the 17th century, immigration led to a four-fold increase in the population of London, most of which took place outside the City. By 1660 the City housed only a quarter of the population. Building spread along the river from the City, through the village of Charing and on to Westminster. It also spread north from the Strand with the development of the Covent Garden piazza and Seven Dials. These newly fashionable areas escaped the Great Fire of 1666, which consumed much of the City.

During the following 150 years, as London continued to expand, Covent Garden passed from being fashionable to being densely populated and deprived. Piecemeal, uncontrolled development led to the creation of numerous courtyards. Drury Lane alone spawned 27 of these insanitary refuges for the poor along the 500 m between Long Acre and the Strand. Particular areas, known as 'rookeries', developed in which housing and living conditions were appalling. The most notorious were St Giles, Seven Dials, The Bermudas (north of the Strand) and Clare Market (near the Aldwych). Such areas posed a threat to the affluent – doctors summoned at night to the British Lying-In Hospital near Seven Dials had sedan chairs provided by the hospital to ensure their safety.

Then, starting in the 1820s, slum clearance programmes began. New roads were driven through the worst areas: William IV and Adelaide Streets cleared The Bermudas (1820s); New Oxford Street cut through St Giles (1847) and Short's Garden through Seven Dials (1850); and Kingsway and Aldwych cleared Clare Market (1905).

Endell Street (1840s) and Charing Cross Road (1864) were built to improve travel between Holborn and the Strand. And in the 1860s Victoria Embankment, containing the new main sewer, contributed to cleaning and redefining the riverbank. There have been few fundamental alterations since then.

While the changing roles of Church, Crown and City are the main theme of this walk, three other themes will be illustrated. One is the competitive nature of health care, in particular between teaching hospitals. Like any other industry, providers of care compete both for income and for status. You will see how three major hospitals and their associated medical schools – King's College, Charing Cross and Westminster – competed in the 19th century.

A second theme is the international nature of health care. Many developments in London have been the result of importing ideas and innovations from abroad. Examples you will encounter include: the first lying-in hospital in England, a direct consequence of the involvement of doctors in childbirth as a result of the importation of obstetric forceps from France; King's College Hospital, where not only nursing, but also hospitals themselves were reformed by religious sisterhoods based on a German model; St Peter's Hospital for Stone, which was the first hospital in England to adopt new surgical methods from the continent that helped establish the specialty of urology; and the Institute of Chinese Medicine, which has led the introduction of acupuncture and other therapies from China.

Finally, look out for the way some health care buildings live on after being abandoned by health care. On this walk, you will see old hospital buildings being used as apartments, a hotel, a club and gallery, and a police station. And a coroner's court and mortuary now houses a nursery school.

The walk starts at Tottenham Court Road underground station. Leave the station by Exit 4, onto New Oxford Street. Turn right and, after 20 m, turn right again. After 40 m cross the road and head along St Giles High Street towards the church of St Giles, surrounded by plane trees. Stop outside the gates to the church.

St Giles High Street, the continuation west of High Holborn, was the principal Roman road running west out of the City, which, as you can see, was forced to curve. This was to avoid a marshy area to the north (the other side of the road). The marshland was eventually drained in the 13th century and converted to pasture. By then, **St Giles Hospital for Lepers** had been established. It was one of ten leper hospitals, each established on one of the roads out of London. Unusually for the time, this one was founded by the Crown, specifically by Matilda, wife of Henry I.

As you face the church, the hospital grounds covered a triangle bordered by St Giles High Street (to your left), Charing Cross Road (to your right) and Shaftesbury Avenue (beyond the church). None of the buildings remains. There was a chapel (on the site of the present church), four spital (hospital) houses (to your

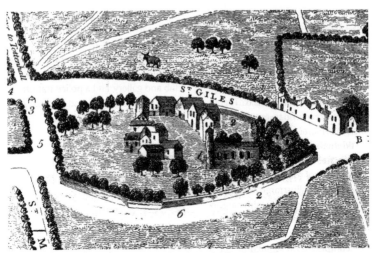

St Giles Hospital, showing the chapel and, on the far right of its extensive grounds, spital houses for leprosy patients

left) to accommodate 40 patients, and the Master's house (towards Charing Cross Road to your right). The rest of the extensive site was farmed by the patients and staff. While nominally for those suffering from leprosy (p. 17), many of those consigned here are likely to have had other skin conditions, indistinguishable at the time from leprosy.

One unique role the hospital fulfilled was to provide a large bowl of ale – St Giles' Bowl – to condemned prisoners being transported from Newgate (a mile away in the City) to the gallows at Tyburn (modern-day Marble Arch). (The original entrance to the churchyard, Resurrection Gate, has been moved to the right of the church in Flitcroft Street.)

Governance of the hospital was contested over several centuries between the Church, Crown and City. An example of the hostility between Crown and Church occurred around 1300. To put St Giles Hospital out of the reach of the Bishop of London, Edward I granted ownership to a religious order from Navarre (northern Spain). This so displeased the Archbishop of Canterbury that he forcibly entered the hospital. A second example, this time of conflict between City and Church, occurred in 1334 when the City, which had the exclusive right to consign lepers to the hospital, discovered that the religious order running the hospital was turning it into a monastery by ousting lepers and installing monks. And another example of conflict between Church and Crown occurred in 1391 when the Bishop of London forced entry with an armed band. This prompted the Crown to give the hospital to the Abbott of St Mary Graces (Tower Hill).

Despite the gradual disappearance of leprosy, the hospital

Leprosy

Leprosy was probably introduced to England by slave labourers of the Roman army. Initially, the Church viewed leprosy as evidence of sinfulness, and the afflicted lost their common law and property rights. From 660, lepers were prohibited from marrying and had to wear distinctive clothing, carry a staff and a warning bell or rattle. Once defined as leprous, victims underwent a 'leper's mass' and were then excluded from their town to become itinerant beggars, with the Church having declared: 'Be thou dead to the world but alive again to God.' At times, far worse events followed the mass, including being burnt at the stake or buried alive. Social status was no protector: in the early 11th century, Aelfward, the Bishop of London, was deemed leprous and was cast out to wander the countryside.

Following the First Crusade (1099), some crusaders returned with leprosy, thus forcing the Church to reinterpret 'having been visited by leprosy' as a sign not of sinfulness but of holiness. It was seen as a 'transitory' state between life and death meaning the sufferer would ascend straight to heaven. Their disfigurement meant they were forced to forgo the love of earthly pleasures.

By the 12th century, when the number of people labelled as 'lepers' peaked, there may have been 10,000 in Britain, although the true number is unknown. As the diagnosis was made by a priest or monk (or even by a watchman, protecting the inhabitants of a town from 'intruders'), it was far from accurate. It covered any 'dirty' condition of the skin including scabies, syphilis, vitiligo, psoriasis or even smallpox. (Indeed, it was

not until 1847 that diagnostic distinctions were made, and not until 1873 that Hansen identified the infectious cause.)

Although a few leper (lazar) houses/ hospitals had been established in the 7th century in England, like other medieval hospitals (p. 35) most were founded between 1100 and 1400, particularly around 1200, outside a city's walls. There were ten around London, each located on one of the main roads out of the City: St Giles, St James, Hackney, Mile End, Kingsland, Holloway, Enfield, Knightsbridge, Hammersmith and Southwark. In 1191 the City took on their supervision. On average, those admitted lived for about ten years. It was seen by some as similar to being consigned to a low holy order. The only benefit lepers enjoyed was the right to beg (denied to others). However, as this encouraged imposters, an ordinance banning lepers from begging in the City of London was passed in 1346.

During the Reformation (1530s), four of London's leper hospitals were dissolved. The six that remained were transferred to the jurisdiction of St Bartholomew's Hospital, although leprosy was soon to disappear from London (1559). The cause of its disappearance is uncertain. Possible explanations include: the great famine of 1315–16 and the Black Death of 1348, killing many sufferers; climate change – cooling in the 13th century led to more clothing being used, reducing the opportunity for transmission; the introduction of TB, which competitively replaced leprosy; a rising standard of living; and more accurate diagnosis.

survived until the Reformation when, in 1539, all but the chapel was demolished. The Palladian-style church you see today, designed by Henry Flitcroft, was built in 1730.

Before entering the churchyard, note the area on the other side of St Giles High Street with new high-rise buildings. In the 18th and 19th centuries, this was the notorious St Giles rookery, an area of poor housing, overcrowding and deprivation. William Hogarth set his painting *Gin Lane* here, reflecting the gin-drinking epidemic of the 1750s. By 1831, 30,000 people, including escaped slaves (referred to at the time as St Giles' Blackbirds), were crammed in. The intended solution, driving New Oxford Street through the heart of the area in 1847, certainly eliminated the slums, although it did little to make the area more inviting.

Walk through the churchyard (to the right of the church) and leave by the gate on the far side into St Giles Passage. After 50 m turn left onto Shaftesbury Avenue and stop after another 30 m opposite a fine red-brick and terracotta building, the **Hôpital et Dispensaire Français**.

The original central, grand entrance has been removed and converted to a window.

In 1861, a French doctor, Achille Vintras, established a dispensary to provide care for French-speaking residents and visitors. In 1867 it became a hospital, initially

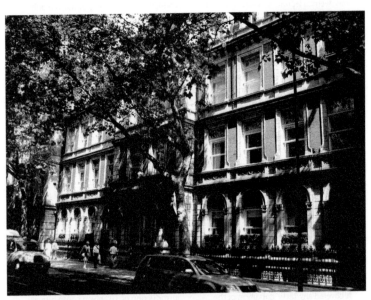

Nouvel Hôpital et Dispensaire Français, built in 1889, which served French-speaking residents and visitors. The original main entrance became a window when it was converted to a hotel

occupying a building near Leicester Square but then moving to these custom-built premises in 1889. This example of health care for foreigners (below) had 50 beds together with a convalescent home in Brighton. The hospital proved so attractive that Soho prostitutes (of all nationalities) drifted away from the Lock Hospital (for venereal disease) in Soho and sought treatment here. It survived until 1966 when lack of finance led to its closure, although an outpatient dispensary has survived, now located in Hammersmith. The building, acquired by the NHS, became the Shaftesbury Hospital, one of four urology hospitals (p. 44) in Covent Garden. All four closed in 1992 when services were transferred to the Middlesex Hospital. The building has since been converted to its current use as the Covent Garden Hotel.

Continue 100 m along Shaftesbury Avenue to the

Health care for foreigners

Since the 18th century, special health care facilities for foreign residents have been established in London: the Scottish Hospital in Blackfriars (1673), the French Huguenot Hospital in St Luke's (1718), the Jew's Hospital in Mile End (1807), the German Hospital in Dalston (1845), the French Dispensary in Fitzrovia (1861), the Italian Hospital in Queen Square (1884), the Institute of Chinese Medicine in Charing Cross (1990), and the Japan Green Medical Centre in St Luke's (1991). Their destinies have been quite varied.

The Scottish Hospital, established because Scots were not entitled to parochial Poor Law assistance or admission to Barts or St Thomas', was run by governors and supported by donations. It closed after seven years when its policy changed to providing outdoor relief.

French Huguenots escaping persecution successfully petitioned the King to be allowed to establish their own hospital, La Providence. Royal approval was on condition that they only accepted French protestants and their descendants, and that patients take the oath of allegiance, supremacy and abjuration. It survived as a hospital until 1865 when it changed to an almshouse and moved to Hackney and then in 1960 to Rochester, Kent.

The Jew's Hospital, Neve Tzeduk, consisted mostly of a boarding school for children, although it also provided nursing care for the frail elderly. The latter only lasted until 1863 when it moved to Norwood. Meanwhile the London Hospital had established two wards and a kosher kitchen with a 'Hebrew Cook' in 1842.

The German Hospital was of great importance in the development of health services in Britain. It was here that Florence Nightingale first encountered nurses trained at the Kaiserwerth Institute in Germany, the model that was to transform nursing and hospitals. After World War II, during which the German staff were interned, the hospital was incorporated into the NHS, finally closing in 1987.

The dispensary established for French-speaking residents and visitors to London expanded after six years to become the Nouvel Hôpital et Dispensaire Français near Leicester Square. It was so successful that it built a fine new hospital in 1889 on Shaftesbury Avenue. It closed in 1966 but the Dispensaire Français survived, moving first to Euston Road and in 2008 to Hammersmith.

In 1884 Giovanni Ortelli, aware of the difficulties experienced by his non-English-speaking compatriots in London's hospitals, donated two properties in Queen Square for the treatment of Italians and Italian-speaking people. However, from the start the Ospedale Italiano also welcomed other people. To ensure the public knew this, the building had as an inscription on its façade: Charity knows no restriction of country. It eventually closed in 1990.

Some immigrant groups brought with them their own traditional medical system that initially served their own community but later provided a service for the wider population. The best example of this has been Chinese medicine during the 20th century. The extent of its impact can be seen in the establishment of clinics and training programmes by bodies such as the Institute of Chinese Medicine in Covent Garden.

The newest service for foreigners is the Japan Green Medical Centre, which provides primary care and diagnostic investigations for Japanese-speaking residents and visitors. Over a third of its patients come from outside the UK, from as far afield as the Middle East and Africa. It has Japanese staff and is run by the Japan Green Hospital company based in Singapore. The centre moved to the City in 2005.

pedestrian crossing, cross the road and turn right into Monmouth Street. If you walk on the left side of the street, you can see the first-floor lettering on the back of the Hôpital Français. On reaching Seven Dials, turn left into Short's Gardens. Cross Neal Street and stop at the next junction, Endell Street.

The area you have just walked through was another infamous rookery in the early 19th century. Endell Street (1840s) and Short's Gardens (1850) were part of the attempt to clear the slums and refashion the area. Despite this,

poverty and hardship remained endemic. Voluntary dispensaries and hospitals were beyond the reach of most residents, as letters of recommendation were needed. The only option was the **St Giles' & St George's Workhouse**, which stood on the other side of Endell Street (now occupied by a modern block of flats to your left, Dudley Court). Built in 1727, the workhouse expanded so that by 1777 it could accommodate 520 people. Despite being the responsibility of the local parishes, the Crown felt some obligation to its poorest citizens.

In the 1820s George IV funded some improvements.

In 1879 a workhouse infirmary (p. 54) was built, but this soon proved insufficient, so in 1895 another much larger infirmary was added: a five-storey grim and forbidding Gothic-style tower named Dudley House (a name retained by the current block of flats). The ground floor accommodated a dispensary providing outpatient care, two floors were dedicated to 'imbeciles', and two floors to those with 'skin conditions'. Although it ceased to be used as a workhouse infirmary in 1914, it reopened in 1915 as a temporary military hospital (p. 250). The Endell Street Military Hospital was run by the newly created Women's Hospital Corps and was the only British hospital ever founded by women for men. By the time it closed in 1920, it had admitted and treated 26,000 men. The building survived until 1978, being used by the post office and the public health laboratory service.

One of the hazards that impoverished women faced was from childbirth (p. 22). Until the middle of the 18th century, the only assistance available was from self-trained midwives who were themselves mostly uneducated women from the poorer classes. Influenced by the development of forceps in France, doctors in London started showing an interest in childbirth in the 1730s. The first hospital with so-called 'man-midwives' (including the leading surgeon, William Hunter) was the Middlesex Hospital in 1745. Following a falling-out with their

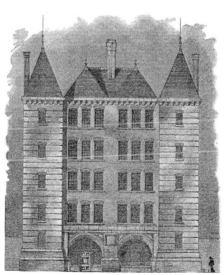

The rather forbidding St Giles' & St George's Workhouse Infirmary (1895) in Short's Gardens, demolished in 1978

medical colleagues, who objected to what they saw as the overuse of beds for childbirth, the 'man-midwives' decided to set up their own lying-in hospital.

The **British Lying-In Hospital for Married Women** was established in 1749 in Brownlow (now Betterton) Street, 50 m to your right along Endell Street. The building has long since been demolished. Women were admitted to the 20 beds in the last month of pregnancy and remained in hospital for three weeks after delivery. Demand was such that patients were selected

Childbirth

Until the 18th century, assistance during childbirth was provided by relatives or by midwives, who were mostly uneducated women from the poorer classes. Formal training of midwives had started in France in the early 16th century, but in England the requirements of a midwife in 1720 were still 'not fat, considerate, grave, patient, pleasant and follows advice'. Houses where midwives could assist women existed but remained unregulated until 1733.

Meanwhile, surgeons were starting to show an interest in childbirth. William Smellie started practising in Pall Mall as a man-midwife (accoucheur), and in 1739 Richard Manningham set up a nursing home for childbirth in Jermyn Street but without medical staff. The few surgeons who did practise midwifery were looked down on by their colleagues, threatened by female midwives and criticised by clerics.

Despite such hostility, concern about the poor outcome of pregnancy among 'the wives of poor, industrious tradesmen, soldiers and sailors' led, in 1745, to the establishment of the first lying-in beds in a voluntary general hospital (p. 148) in London, the Middlesex Hospital. Two years later, the man-midwives,

who included William Hunter, left and established the first hospital to specialise in obstetrics, the British Lying-In Hospital in Covent Garden. This was followed by the establishment of several more, including the City of London, the General (which evolved from Manningham's nursing home and later became Queen Charlotte's Hospital), and the Westminster. Women's privacy was literally guarded by doormen in livery, and visiting by family members was very limited. Initially, at least, these were patriarchal institutions that not only undermined female midwives, but also took control of childbirth from women. Despite this, they introduced formal training for midwives.

The vast majority of babies, however, continued to be delivered at home or in a workhouse. To provide some assistance, Lying-in Institutions were established that provided domiciliary midwifery. General hospitals showed no interest. After the Middlesex Hospital closed its lying-in beds in 1786, apart from a short-lived lying-in ward in King's College Hospital in the 1860s, there was no provision until the Royal Free Hospital established a service in 1918.

The number of man-midwives increased rapidly through the late 18th and the 19th centuries as midwifery became an essential component of medical education. It was not until 1881 that female midwives organised themselves to meet the growing encroachment by male doctors. Despite resistance from doctors, who saw it as a threat to their livelihoods, midwives were successful when, in 1902, the Midwives' Act recognised their role and made it illegal for unqualified midwives to practise. Their position was further strengthened when the 1911 National Insurance Act established the right for married women to choose between a midwife and a doctor attending their delivery. During the first half of the 20th century, many births took place at home or in Maternity Homes run by midwives, but as hospital obstetric departments developed under the NHS, the place of birth shifted.

randomly by drawing coloured balls from a bag. On leaving they had to 'give thanks' and were quizzed by the governors on their views of the quality of their care – a level of concern rarely achieved today. Despite such an exemplary approach, the hospital attracted criticism in 1751 when a 'Petition of the Unborn Babe' was sent to the Royal

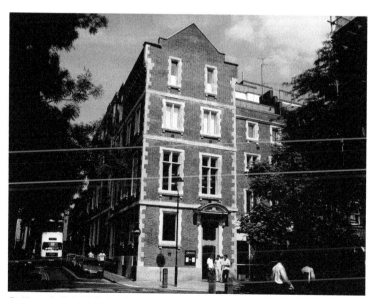

Built as the British Lying-In Hospital in 1845, it was subsequently home to St Paul's Hospital from 1921 to 1992

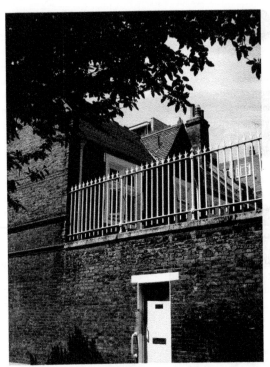

Macklin Street entrance to the secluded St Giles' & St George's Almshouses, built in 1885 although located here since 1783

College of Physicians claiming that 'experiments' were leading to the deaths of mothers and babies. This proved to be no more than a minor irritation to the governors, and in the 1840s, when the creation of Endell Street provided the opportunity to expand, a new hospital was built. The Jacobean-style red-brick building that you can see diagonally across the road (No. 24, now housing a private club) served as the lying-in hospital until 1913, when it moved to Woolwich to merge with the Home for Mothers and Babies.

After its use as a military hospital during World War I, the building became home in 1921 to **St Paul's Hospital for Diseases of the Genito-Urinary Organs and Skin**. St Paul's had been established in Red Lion Square in 1897 by Dr Felix Vinrace, despite opposition from a neighbour who was a Member of Parliament and thought reference to genito-urinary diseases in the inscription above the hospital door was indecent. While public recognition and acceptance of genito-urinary diseases in general, and venereal diseases (p. 123) in particular, was limited, the level of need was considerable. Despite such high demand, the hospital

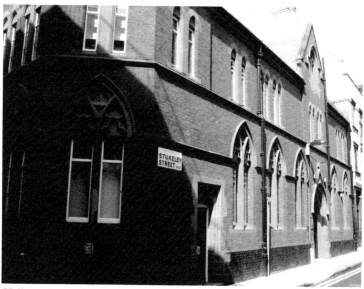

Holborn Coroner's Court and Mortuary (1883). The entrance to the court was to the right, and the entrance to the upstairs mortuary on the left. It closed in the 1950s

sought to develop its more specialist urology service, reflecting its close relationship with the leading urology hospital, St Peter's. This culminated in a merger in 1948 when both were incorporated into the NHS.

Cross Endell Street and continue along Short's Gardens. The site of the old workhouse infirmary (on your left) is still associated with health care – the Covent Garden Medical Centre provides primary care for local residents. At the end turn left into Drury Lane and stop after 30 m opposite Stukeley Street. In the 17th century, the street was lined with overcrowded, dilapidated houses. It was in a house here (on the left, now a hotel entrance) that the Great Plague of 1665, which

killed 56,000 people, is believed to have started when a group of Flemish weavers opened imported goods from Holland.

Walk down Stukeley Street and, after about 100 m, right into Smart's Place. At the end on the left is the entrance to **St Giles' & St George's Almshouses**, another example of parish provision. Originally located on High Holborn, they were relocated here in 1783 and rebuilt in 1885. You can see little of the 13 houses around their cramped L-shaped courtyard. The changing environs mean that a visitor's description in 1892, of 'cheerless homes … in this foul cul-de-sac', no longer holds true.

Return to Stukeley Street, turn right and follow the road round to the right to where it meets Macklin Street. If you look to the right along Macklin Street, you will see, about 50 m along on the right, some white railings on top of a high brick wall. This is the other entrance to the almshouses.

The red-brick Gothic-style building on the corner in front of you was the **Holborn Coroner's Court and Mortuary**, built in 1883. Although coroners' duties are now largely confined to investigating the cause of any sudden, unexpected or unnatural deaths, coroners (originally 'crowners') were established by the Crown in the 12th century to ensure that taxes and other funds were not stolen by corrupt sheriffs, despite the latter also being officers of the Crown! The coroners' role was to investigate all violent and unexplained deaths to ensure that the revenue from fines imposed on murderers by the courts found its way into the Crown's coffers. Nowadays, coroners are usually lawyers, although some are doctors. Inquests were held on the ground floor of this building with the mortuary above. Although the court closed in 1910, the mortuary was used until the 1950s.

Walk along the pedestrianised section of Macklin Street, and at the end turn right into Newton Street. Take the first left (Parker Street) and then right, along Kingsway. After 20 m cross over and walk straight ahead down Remnant Street into Lincoln's Inn Fields. This square was at the heart of medical London during the early decades of the 19th century when doctors moved

here from Moorfields (modern-day Finsbury Circus and Square). Houses were first built here in the 1640s, despite opposition from lawyers on the far side of the square in Lincoln's Inn, but it is now a hotch-potch of 18th, 19th and 20th century houses, mansion blocks and office blocks.

Cross over and enter the gardens in the centre of the square. Head to the right through the gardens. Halfway along you can see to your right, across the road, two fine Palladian-style houses (Nos 57 and 58) with a shared entrance. In the 1820s and 30s, the one on the left was the home of one of the leading medical societies (p. 184), the **Royal Society of Medicine**. Carry on to the corner of the gardens where you will see a bronze bust of John Hunter, the 18th century founder of modern surgery. Continue on round and take the next exit, in front of the neo-classical **Royal College of Surgeons**.

The College owes its existence to both the City and the Crown. In 1540 the City Company of Barber-Surgeons was recognised by Henry VIII when two organisations that represented those performing surgery, the Company of Barbers and the much smaller Fellowship of Surgeons, merged. They erected a Hall near Aldersgate where they maintained an uneasy collaboration for 200 years. By the mid-18th century, the surgeons sought independence, and in 1745 the Crown recognised a separate Company of Surgeons. They built their own Hall near Newgate Prison, the source of criminals' bodies for dissection.

The move here in 1800 was prompted partly by surgeons' pursuit of the rich, upper classes on whom doctors depended for their income, and partly because Surgeons' Hall could not accommodate the newly acquired bequest from John Hunter of his vast museum of anatomical specimens. At the same time, the Company became a royal college (p. 194), giving surgeons similar status to that of physicians.

Initially, the College occupied No. 41, one of the fine houses that lined this side of the square. Having acquired a neighbouring house, the first Royal College building on this site was erected in 1813. Designed by George Dance the Younger, it had a neo-classical portico including the six large fluted Ionic columns you can see today. Following the acquisition of two more houses, Charles Barry expanded and remodelled the building in 1836. But the changes did not end there. Throughout the 19th century, changes were made, including the unsympathetic addition by Stephen Salter of two storeys, one with wreathed circular windows.

The building suffered badly during World War II, with half the 60,000 specimens in the museum destroyed. Reconstruction plus the addition of the Nuffield College of Surgical Sciences (to the left of the main building) was not completed until 1957. The latter provided accommodation for foreign postgraduate students, reflecting the increasingly international role of an organisation that had started as a City guild. Until 1996, it also housed the Institute of Basic Medical Research, one of the postgraduate

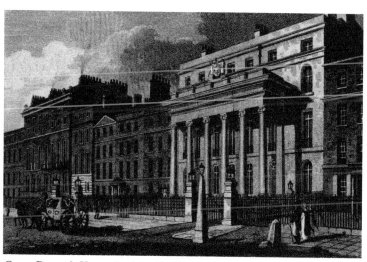

George Dance the Younger's original building for the Royal College of Surgeons (1813), set amid terraced houses, since when it has been repeatedly modified

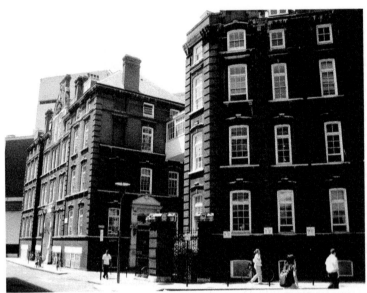

The two interconnected wings of the Strand Union Workhouse Infirmary (1903), which subsequently became a public hospital for women with venereal disease (1919–52) and then a urology hospital (until 1992). It was demolished in 2011

institutes (p. 201) of the University of London.

Unlike the situation in the 19th century when the museum was only open to surgeons, aristocrats and foreign dignitaries (as it was felt inappropriate for members of the middle and lower classes to view the contents), the Hunterian Museum, recently beautifully remodelled, is open (free) to all members of the public (www.rcseng.ac.uk/museums).

Cross over to the College and walk to the right. Until 2015 the neighbouring building houses the **Research Institute of Cancer Research UK**. This organisation was formed in 2002 by the merger of two charities, the Imperial Cancer Research Fund and the Cancer Research Campaign. The former, the first cancer research organisation in Britain, was established in 1902, soon after the introduction of the first effective anti-cancer treatment, radium. The first home of its research laboratories was the Conjoint Examination Hall on Victoria Embankment (which you will visit later). After several moves, the site here became available as a result of World War II bombing. The undistinguished building you see opened in 1963, since when it has been extended twice. It houses about 30 research groups funded by public donations. In 2015 it is due to move to the Crick Institute by St Pancras station.

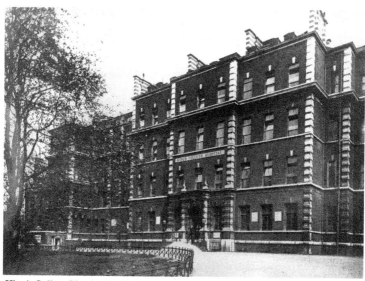

King's College Hospital, built in 1860, replaced the disused workhouse in which the hospital had been established in 1840. When the hospital moved to south London in 1913, the building was demolished

Continue and turn left into Portsmouth Street. The Old Curiosity Shop on the left gives an idea of housing in the mid-17th century (rather than 1567, as claimed). Opposite it stood the **Strand Union Workhouse Infirmary**. Constructed in 1903, it was sold to the Metropolitan Asylums Board (p. 179) in 1919 to accommodate a hospital for treating venereal disease, a problem that had not been adequately recognised until its toll became apparent during World War I. The Board established the Institution for Venereal Diseases with 52 beds for women. In 1930, when the Board's responsibilities were taken over by the London County Council, it was given the less stigmatising name of Sheffield Street Hospital, although its role did not alter.

It became part of the NHS and was renamed again in 1952, as St Philip's Hospital, to distance it even further from its workhouse origins. Also, its remit broadened to include other genito-urinary conditions, influenced by its collaboration with two urology hospitals, St Paul's and St Peter's. By 1969 the focus was on renal (kidney) diseases. Along with the other urology hospitals, it moved to the Middlesex Hospital in 1992. The building was acquired by the London School of Economics (LSE) in 1992, which proceeded to demolish it in 2011 as part of its redevelopment of the area.

Walk on along Portsmouth Street as far as Portugal Street. The large red-brick building on the opposite side of the street (now the LSE Library) was built in 1920 as the headquarters and distribution centre of the newsagents WH Smith & Son. It occupies the original site of **King's College Hospital**.

Having failed in the 1830s to persuade the recently established Charing Cross Hospital to provide clinical experience for its medical students, King's College (on the Strand) was forced to make other arrangements. It acquired and renovated a disused workhouse that had been built on this site in 1771. King's College Hospital opened in 1840 and soon boasted 120 beds, for which Mrs Ward, the matron, had six nurses and seven helpers. Their lack of training and skills was increasingly of concern to the governors, although it was no worse than for other voluntary general hospitals (p. 148) in London. In an historic move in 1856, the nursing service was taken over by the Anglican nursing sisterhood (p. 163) of St John's House, the first major 'contracting-out' of a hospital activity in the UK. Of even greater importance, it heralded the transformation of hospitals from places of danger to the citadels of healing they were to become in the 20th century.

Despite significant improvements, the limitations of the old workhouse buildings were apparent. They were gradually replaced, such that by 1860 there was a grand 200-bedded hospital built on sanitarian principles. It included an operating theatre, which accommodated 300 students, and a chapel accommodating 200, reflecting the hospital's religious commitment. Although the new nursing regime led to major improvements, it created considerable hostility among medical staff as the matron demanded more nurses and greater independence. In 1874 the sisterhood's refusal to compromise led to some governors resigning. This harmed the hospital's ability to attract medical students (a key source of income for their honorary physicians and surgeons). Despite attracting the famous surgeon Joseph Lister to the staff in 1877, the resentment of doctors and managers persisted, culminating in the curtailment of the contract with St John's House in 1884. In contrast to the old regime, the new matron, Miss Monk (known as Sister Kitty), held that nurses should be loyal and helpful handmaids to the doctors and saw nursing as a vocation, not a profession.

The religious foundations of the hospital were tempered in 1903 when the requirement for staff and students to make a religious declaration, undergo a test and attend chapel daily were lifted. However, morning and evening prayers were still being read daily in the chapel by the matron in 1935. By then the hospital had moved to Denmark Hill in south London (in 1913), encouraged both by the family of WH Smith (a major benefactor of the hospital, who wanted the land here for their company) and one of its main funders, the King's Fund, which sought the migration of some central London hospitals to the suburbs. This illustrates how, even in the 20th century, the Crown (which played an active role in the King's Fund) was still influencing health care in London.

Standing here in the 1880s, you would have seen the grand front of the four-storey hospital set at a 30-degree angle to the street. And you may have glimpsed Foreman, the tall burly and domineering hall porter who extracted a shilling from each student to pay for planting the flower bed in front of the hospital.

Turn right into Portugal Street, cross over and take the second on the left, Clare Market. In the 18th and early 19th centuries, this was the heart of another 'rookery'. In 1831 over 42,000 people lived in a quarter of a square mile, struggling to survive in slum housing. This was one reason King's College elected to site its hospital in the area. As with other rookeries, the solution was to drive major new roads through to stimulate redevelopment. In this case, Kingsway and Aldwych were created in 1905.

Turn right into Houghton Street, and when you reach Aldwych turn right towards Kingsway. Cross half of Kingsway, and then go left across Aldwych to Bush House. Walk about 100 m to the right and then left along India Place to the Strand. Cross over and enter Somerset House.

Walk across the extensive courtyard and through the building on the far side to the riverside terrace beyond. Turn left and walk 100 m along the terrace as far as the large archway in the façade. The building beyond the archway on the right was the original home of King's College, whose establishment was a fine example of collaboration between the Church, Crown and City. It was founded in 1830 in response to the establishment of the secular, godless University College in 1828 (which in turn had been a response to the exclusion of non-Anglicans from Oxford and Cambridge universities). A committee, led by the Prime Minister (the Duke of Wellington), was committed to establishing a college that would put Protestantism firmly back on the curriculum. George IV agreed to be patron. Students would have to be Anglican and undertake religious studies as part of their training.

As will be apparent, the college building, designed by Robert Smirke, formed the east wing of Somerset House. If you look through the archway, you can see the original three-storey building on the right, with giant Corinthian pilasters above the central entrance. It was extended in 1886 and again in 1932. **King's College Medical School** occupied the river-end of this building. The ground-floor rooms housed the anatomy department, and the upper floors provided residences for medical students. The medical school moved to south London with the hospital in 1915.

In the early 19th century, medical education was obtained in private anatomy schools (p. 128) and by apprenticeship with physicians and surgeons in the voluntary hospitals.

Gradually, the large voluntary general hospitals established their own medical schools (largely as a source of income), leading to the demise of the private schools by the middle of the century. There were two exceptions to this pattern. Although university education in England for medical practitioners had been confined to Oxford and Cambridge, in 1828 University College, and two years later King's College, established a medical school, thus posing a threat to the voluntary hospitals' endeavours to establish their own medical schools. That was why nearby Charing Cross Hospital rejected King's College's approaches in the 1830s.

Walk back along the terrace in front of Somerset House. Up until the 1530s, this bank of the river from the City to Westminster was lined by fine episcopal palaces and mansions. River access was more important (and more comfortable) than road access by the Strand. Before construction of the Victoria Embankment in the late 19th century (which you can see if you look over the balustrade), boats and barges could sail into the wharfs below the terrace you are on. During the Reformation, property was transferred by the Crown from clerics to noblemen. One, the Duke of Somerset, swept away five small palaces to make way for Somerset House. In turn, after 1660, most of the grandees' palaces were demolished, this being the one exception.

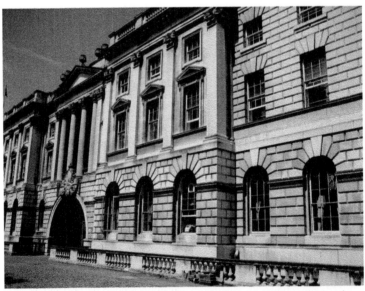

Robert Smirke's addition to Somerset House in 1830 formed its east wing (to the right of the archway) and was the home of King's College Medical School until 1915

At the end go up the ramp onto Lancaster Place. Descend the steps on your left to the Embankment. Turn right, cross over into Savoy Place and stop in front of the Institution of Electrical Engineers. This was designed by Stephen Salter and Percy Adams for the two medical royal colleges as their **Conjoint Examination Hall**. It opened in 1899, some 15 years after the Colleges had instituted their Conjoint Exam for qualifications to practise medicine (LRCP, MRCS). Excess space in the building was leased to the Imperial Cancer Research Fund for research laboratories, and to the Metropolitan Asylums Board for offices. However, somewhat strangely, within a few years the Colleges were prepared to move to another custom-built home in Queen Square, presumably for financial reasons. The façade was altered and an extra storey added in the 1950s.

Continue along Savoy Place and turn right up Savoy Hill. Follow the road to the right where you will see the Queen's Chapel of the Savoy. This is all that remains of one of the greatest 16th century buildings in London and the largest hospital in Britain before 1680, the **Savoy Hospital**. Commissioned by Henry VII and opened in 1517, it was modelled on Santa Maria Nuovo in Florence. It was cruciform in design with an infirmary in the 280 foot main nave (known as the Great Dormitory and divided into

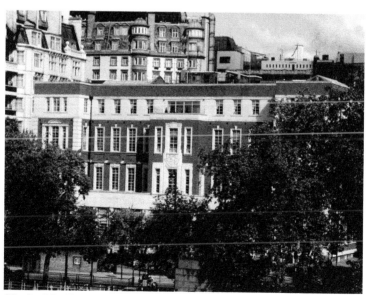

The Conjoint Examination Hall built in 1899 for the two royal colleges (physicians and surgeons) but sold after only ten years to the Institution of Electrical Engineers, which added a storey

12 bays), and private cubicles in the north and south transepts (with a combined length of 200 feet). The nave ran east from where you are standing, along Savoy Hill and on towards Somerset House.

Every evening poor men were received and 100 selected for admission for the night. Only the sick were allowed to remain during the day. Those admitted proceeded to one of the three chapels to pray and were then allocated a bed in the dormitory. Baths and clean clothes were provided. There was a master, four chaplains, two priests, four altarists (to assist in services), seven servants, a matron and 12 sisters (who had to be over 36 and unmarried). Everyone wore a blue uniform with a red and gold Tudor rose on the breast. Patients were tended by a physician, a surgeon and an apothecary, two of whom were paid for by the Crown. This was the first London hospital to provide medical practitioners. To what extent

this was an advantage, given the repeated purging, blood-letting and noxious potions administered, is debatable. The hospital was seen to have outlived its usefulness by 1702, although the buildings survived until a fire destroyed them in 1776. All that remains is the small chapel you are standing beside.

Retrace your steps down Savoy Hill to Savoy Place, turn right and after 40 m cross over and enter Victoria Embankment Gardens, created when the embankment was constructed in the 1860s. Take the path to the right, and after 200 m take the right fork in the path. Note the large monolithic building through the trees up to your right. In 1768 this was the site of the Adelphi, one of the first attempts at developing an extensive residential area. It was the creation of the Adam brothers, foremost architects of their day. Through a series of arched vaults, they constructed a platform on this steep riverside site for a

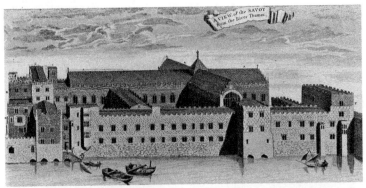

The Savoy Hospital (1517) seen from the river. All that survives is the Savoy Chapel, which can be seen (top left) located at the western end of the main cruciform hospital building

magnificent ensemble of houses. Most of the buildings were wantonly destroyed in 1936, although you can see a few that remain, to the left of the soulless monolithic replacement.

One of the more dubious original residents was James Graham, who established a **Temple of Health (or Hymen)** to combat infertility. For 50 guineas a night he provided a 'celestial bed' complete with eastern perfumes, soft music and bacchic dances, which he claimed would rejuvenate couples and promote conception. A less dubious service that was also housed in the Adelphi was a sea-water bath where the supposed medicinal benefits could be obtained without having to travel to the coast.

Continue along the right-hand path and you will come to the one surviving water-gate, which each of the riverside palaces had before the embankment was built. It was built in 1675 for York House. An information board provides more details of its history.

If you were to continue along the river you would go under Charing Cross railway station. Immediately beyond was, for 315 years, the site of a medieval hospital (p. 35), **St Mary Rounceval**. It was founded in 1229 as a convent for a priory in Rouncevaux, Navarre (in the Pyrenees). This was at a time when religious orders extended across Europe like modern multinational companies. At times, this created tension with the other principal power, the Crown. During the reign of Henry V, England was at war with France, so foreign institutions were taken over by the Crown. St Mary's was granted to a more subservient English order in 1478 and survived until the Reformation, when, in 1544, like other church institutions, the hospital was dissolved. No contemporary illustrations survive but it is recorded that the site was surrounded by a lime-washed mud wall and there was a great gate on to the Strand. The chapel was alongside the river, the infirmary was on the far side of the site, and the rest of the estate was a garden.

Returning to more recent times, on a summer's afternoon in 1908 you would have found over 2,000 nurses,

Medieval hospitals

Although military hospitals existed during the Roman occupation, the next clear account of hospitals is not until 1070. Between 1070 and 1150, 68 spital houses were established in England, providing hospitality (shelter and care) for travellers (particularly for the sick making pilgrimages to centres of healing such as Canterbury). Run by monks or nuns, the better ones provided nourishment, herbal medications and nursing care. Their principal purpose was not the care of the sick per se, but the service of God through promoting spiritual health. Given that physical suffering was seen as a punishment for sin, it was first necessary to make a full confession to the 'physicians of the soul', the priests. The role of patients was to pray for the souls of others, in particular the hospital's rich benefactors, as the passage of the soul through purgatory would be hastened by the intercessionary prayers of the living.

By 1300 there were nine hospitals in London, seven of which were outside the city walls. The basic requirements were a chapel and an infirmary hall, in close proximity so that the bedridden could 'benefit' from the religious devotions. Often it was a single building in which patients occupied the nave and the chancel acted as the chapel. Unlike large institutions elsewhere in Europe, there was little or no involvement on the part of physicians, surgeons or apothecaries (until the Savoy Hospital in 1517). Heads of hospitals were well paid, raising funds by selling indulgences and enhancing their popularity as a healing centre by acquiring religious relics. Many hospitals specialised: for the mentally retarded, blind, crippled, or, most commonly, for leprosy (p. 17).

By the end of the 14th century, there was growing criticism: the Crown was concerned about the 50–60 hospitals that were under foreign control, and the Lollards accused the clergy of misappropriating funds. Lollards advocated that religious hospitals in England be replaced by 100 new ones under lay control (the first recorded proposal for national planning).

In the 15th century, nursing standards were thought to be declining due to a lack of vocation, and patients were often badly treated by the brethren (including illicit consorting in the kitchen!). Mismanagement, financial problems and corruption were rife. By the end of the century, Henry VII decided to establish three large hospitals (London, Coventry and York), although only the Savoy Hospital in London was constructed. As a result, London had four 'general' hospitals, all situated outside the city walls: St Mary without Bishopsgate (east), The Savoy (west), St Bartholomew's (north) and St Thomas' (south).

Pressure for reform continued. By the time of the Reformation (1530s), there were about 600 hospitals in England. Although the larger hospitals were indistinguishable from monasteries, they were not the intended target of the Reformation. However, all were dissolved, although hospital chapels were often retained and converted into parish churches. The City quickly recognised the need for civic authorities to assume responsibility, and in 1538 the Crown refounded five 'royal' hospitals to be administered by the Corporation of London: St Bartholomew's, St Thomas', St Mary of Bethlehem (later known as Bethlem or Bedlam), the Bridewell (for the idle and unemployed) and Christ's Hospital (for orphans). Later, in 1556, the Savoy Hospital was re-established, the last 'new' hospital until after the Restoration in 1660.

in uniform, here in the gardens. They were here to greet the King and Queen before the royal couple proceeded through the water-gate to open the new home of the Royal National Pension Fund for Nurses (about which, more in a moment). Unlike royalty, walk around the gate and leave the gardens, entering Buckingham Street.

The first building on the right, a modern office block, is on a site that is important in the history of health care for two reasons. First, in the 1880s, a room in one of the houses on the site was home to a fledgling organisation, the **Matrons' Aid Society,** which 66 years later was to become the Royal College of Midwives. It had been founded by two midwives, Zepherina Veitch and Louisa Hubbard, to meet the encroachment by male doctors into care during childbirth. They met resistance not only from doctors, but also from rival nursing organisations. In 1890 the Society sought more space and moved across the street to No. 12 where it remained until 1933. Despite opposition, Parliament passed the Midwives Act in 1902 that established midwifery as an independent profession.

The second connection with health care relates to that royal visit in 1908. Until the 1880s, nurses had no entitlement to a pension, although some of the larger voluntary hospitals provided one for long-serving staff to discourage them from leaving to undertake private work. A key advocate of pensions for nurses, the leading hospital reformer Henry Burdett had

been shocked to learn of the fate of Nurse Steer, who contracted typhus from a patient at the Seamen's Hospital and was so debilitated she was unable to continue nursing. She ended up spending the rest of her life in a workhouse. In 1887 Burdett organised a meeting at the Royal Society for Arts (just round the corner from here) at which the **National Pension Fund for Nurses** was launched. Support was far from universal: Nightingale felt that pensions would increase the cost of nursing to such an extent that hospitals would reduce staffing levels, and hospital governors felt it should be left to them to decide. Despite this, in 1908 the Fund moved to custom-built premises here, Burdett House, which had replaced the two townhouses. Although many nurses deserted the Fund when state pensions were introduced in 1911, it had helped to establish nurses' rights to a pension.

There is one further health care connection in this street. As you walk up Buckingham Street note the last house on the right, home of the leading British orthopaedic journal. Turn right into John Adam Street and walk as far as George Court on the left. Looking ahead, you can make out the raised area created by the Adam brothers to support the terraces of fine houses, including the Royal Society for Arts on the left, with its fluted pilasters and pediment. Across the end of the street is the stunning Adam House, which from 1926 until 1987 housed the leading medical journal, *The Lancet.* The charmless building on the right-hand side, on the site of what had been the centrepiece of the Adelphi, has since 1997 housed the global headquarters of **Smith & Nephew**. Now a leading provider of surgical dressings, endoscopes and joint prostheses, the company was established in 1896 by a dispensing chemist in Hull, Thomas Smith, and his nephew.

Turn down George Court and emerge on the Strand opposite Zimbabwe House, designed by Percy Adams and built of grey Cornish granite and Portland stone for the **British Medical Association**

(BMA). Opened in 1907, it replaced the two houses on the site that the BMA had occupied since 1886. Around the second-floor windows, you can see what remain of several nude statues sculptured by Jacob Epstein. They were denounced at the time in a London paper as outrages against decency and good taste, not the usual basis of criticism of the doctors' trades union. Their current forlorn state is due to erosion rather than attacks by the outraged. The BMA stayed only 16 years before moving to Tavistock Square.

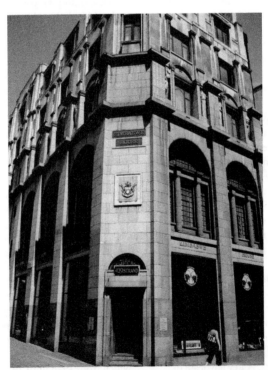

Percy Adams' building for the British Medical Association (1907), with Jacob Epstein's weathered statues around the second-floor windows (now Zimbabwe House)

Cross the Strand. The large, cream-coloured building ahead of you is the old **Charing Cross Hospital**. Designed by Decimus Burton, it opened in 1834. However, the origins of the hospital go back to 1818 when the founder Benjamin Golding, an idealistic young doctor, established a small infirmary on the far side of Trafalgar Square. This then moved to Villiers Street (beside modern-day Charing Cross station) in 1823, where he included a medical school, albeit with only four students. By the time of the move here to Agar Street, this had risen to 22.

His choice of location reflected his commitment to helping the poor, for the surrounding area was another rookery known as The Bermudas (later known as Cribbee Islands). The original building by Burton extended the length of Agar Street but was only 52 feet deep. Most of the rest of the triangular site behind the hospital was occupied by houses. Despite making such impressive progress, Golding had reason to feel threatened. First, in the 1820s, Westminster Hospital toyed with moving from St James's to Charing Cross, and second, in the 1830s, King's College sought to monopolise medical training in the area by inviting Charing Cross Hospital to become its teaching hospital. Golding's resistance led, as you have seen, to King's College having to establish its own hospital.

In 1866 the decision by King's College Hospital to contract out

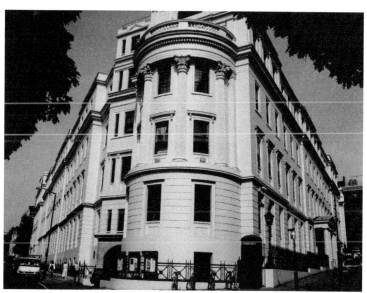

Decimus Burton's original Charing Cross Hospital (1834) can be seen on the right, along Agar Street, although the fourth floor and entrance portico were added in the 1880s. Its subsequent expansion can be seen to the left

nursing to the St John's House nursing sisterhood was copied by Charing Cross Hospital. As with experiences at King's, the arrangement broke down in the 1880s in the face of opposition from doctors and subscribers. When the sisterhood was replaced, the new matron was known as 'Dame of the Wards', a term that was not widely adopted.

Between 1880 and 1902, the hospital enlarged to occupy almost all the land behind it, and the entrance portico you see today was added. Like other voluntary general hospitals, it struggled financially. However, World War I came to its aid. Payments from the Ministry of War restored its financial health, although it remained dependent on the Crown: 13% of the income in 1920 came from the King's Fund. The financial situation was not helped by the matron, Miss Cochrane (known as Cockles), successfully negotiating a day off a week for her nurses, seen as radical at the time, but a move that all London hospitals were forced to copy.

By 1936 the need for a larger site was accepted. First the Adelphi was considered but proved too costly. Instead, with the approval of the King's Fund, a staggering 800 small properties in St Giles (where this walk started) were purchased, but before construction could start World War II intervened. After the war, government policy favoured huge 1,000-bedded hospitals in the suburbs. So the St Giles properties were sold (at a profit)

and attention shifted to Northwick Park in Harrow. However, this move was stymied in 1955 when the University of London suddenly withdrew its support, arguing that it was too far from the rest of the university. Finally, in 1973, despite local opposition to 'an intruder', Charing Cross Hospital moved to a new building on the site of Fulham Hospital in west London.

Initially, the old hospital building was used as a hostel for the destitute and homeless, but it was acquired by the Metropolitan Police in 1974.

As you walk along King William IV Street to your left, look out for the foundation stone on the curved end of Burton's 1834 building and the 'CCH' initials in the railings.

The building at the end of the street on the right was the **Royal Westminster Ophthalmic Hospital.** To get a better view, cross to the other side of King William IV Street. The Infirmary for Diseases of the Eye was established by George Guthrie in 1816 near St Giles Church, one of several eye hospitals (p. 59) established in 19th century London. The building in front of you (now called Apex House) was founded in 1831, three months before that for Charing Cross Hospital. The hospital gained royal recognition in 1854, something that hospitals still seek and value today. It remained here for 86 years before moving to High Holborn in 1926, where, in 1946, it merged with the Central London and the Royal London Ophthalmic Hospitals, eventually becoming part of Moorfields Eye

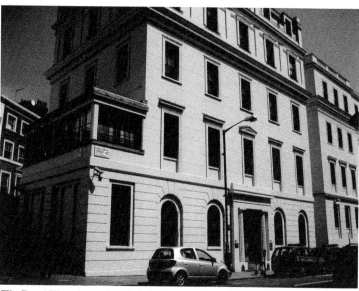

The Royal Westminster Ophthalmic Hospital (1831) until 1926, when the building was incorporated into Charing Cross Hospital, on the right

Hospital. Following its departure, this building was incorporated into Charing Cross Hospital in the late 1920s.

Cross back over King William IV Street into Chandos Place, where you can see the eye hospital's foundation stone. On the other side of Chandos Place is the **Institute of Chinese Medicine**. Established in 1990, its existence in the heart of London reflects both the presence of a local Chinese community and contemporary Western interest in Chinese (and other) traditional methods of healing. As well as providing treatment using acupuncture, herbal medicine, Tui Na and exercise, the staff provide training for Western doctors who

want to incorporate these methods into their practice.

Walk along Chandos Place past the old hospital buildings on your right. Note how the old ophthalmic hospital was attached to Charing Cross Hospital by a second-floor bridge when incorporated in the 1920s. Just after, you will see an arched entrance that was originally for the nurses' home, built in 1902, and meant that the resident nurses no longer had to enter and leave their 'home' via the hospital. In the 1880s, this street (and the two others beside the hospital) was paved with wood blocks to reduce the noise of horse-drawn transport. The 1880s also saw the opening of a new medical school building on the left side at 63 Chandos Street (recently

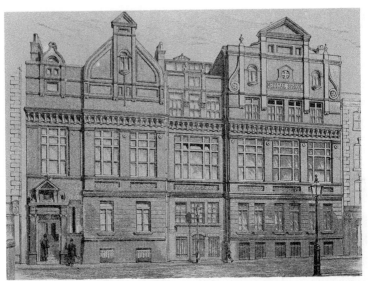

Charing Cross Hospital Medical School (1881) in Chandos Place moved with the hospital to Fulham in 1973, and the building was later demolished

demolished). This was connected to the hospital by a tunnel in order to avoid transporting corpses via the street to the post-mortem room in the school.

At the end of Chandos Place, turn left into Bedford Street and then right into Henrietta Street. Stop after about 50 m outside No. 15, opposite a Queen Anne-style red-brick building containing four shops and a projecting central entrance. The date of its construction, 1882, can be seen above the central second-floor window, and the initials of its original occupant – SPHS – below that window. Crossed keys, the symbol of St Peter, are carved over the main entrance. This was

St Peter's Hospital for Stone until 1992, when, with the three other urology hospitals, it moved to the Middlesex Hospital.

It had been established in 1860 in Marylebone as the Hospital for the Treatment of Stone and Urinary Diseases, the first hospital specialising in this field. It soon acquired a saint's name, consistent with the fashion of the time. Demand from patients meant more space was needed. In 1873, the governors got lucky – an unknown benefactor walked in and presented a sealed packet on the understanding it was not to be opened until he had left. It turned out to contain £10,000. Such an act of generosity made

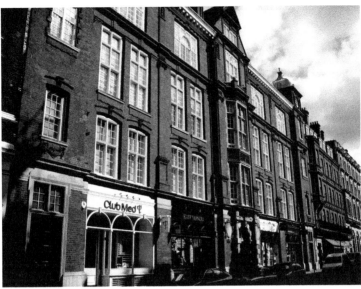

St Peter's Hospital for Stone (1882), with oriel windows above the central entrance and ground-floor shops as an extra source of income. The hospital left in 1992, and the building was converted to apartments

the editor of the *British Medical Journal* apoplectic. He viewed specialist hospitals as unnecessary 'mischievous excrescences on our system of hospital charity' and criticised the benefactor for 'perpetuating an evil'.

The result was the purpose-built premises you see now, including four shops to generate rental income. In the event, demand was such that the space occupied by the shops was needed by the hospital. Further expansion was achieved by acquiring a house, No. 10 opposite the hospital, for a nurses' home (p. 151). In 1948

the hospital was incorporated into the NHS, merging its management with that of St Paul's Hospital, and in 1954 the University of London established its postgraduate institute for urology in No. 10. Since the hospital's departure in 1992, the building has been converted to seven spacious apartments and shops have reoccupied the ground floor.

Continue along Henrietta Street into Covent Garden piazza. Turn left, cross the piazza and leave by James Street. Covent Garden underground station, where the walk ends, is 100 m on the left.

Urology hospitals

'Cutting for stone' (removal of stones from the bladder) was one of the few surgical operations undertaken before the introduction of general anaesthesia in 1846. Not surprisingly, the reputation of a surgeon was, to some extent, dependent on the speed with which he conducted the procedure. The availability of anaesthesia was timely given the doubling in the reported number of deaths from urinary diseases in the 1850s, an observation that some have ascribed to an epidemic of stones resulting from the nutritional deprivations of the 1840s (the so-called 'hungry forties').

The increased demand for surgery contributed to the establishment in 1860 of a voluntary specialist hospital (p. 119), the Hospital for the Treatment of Stone and Urinary Diseases in Great Marylebone Street (now New Cavendish Street). It remained there for only three years before moving to Berners Street and changing its name to St Peter's Hospital for Stone. When it moved in 1882 to custom-built premises in Covent Garden, the editor of the *British Medical Journal*, a critic of specialist hospitals, was apoplectic:

'This institution is one ... of the unnecessary special hospitals which constitute mischievous excrescences on our system of hospital charity; and the ill-advised munificence which endows it only tends to perpetuate an evil which might

otherwise have been expected to die out with those who promoted it.'

This, however, failed to prevent the establishment of additional specialist hospitals. In 1897 Dr Felix Vinrace established a hospital 'For Skin and Genito-Urinary Diseases' in Red Lion Square. With only six beds, it was largely a dispensary treating venereal disease (p. 123). The need for more space led to a move to the abandoned British Lying-In Hospital in Endell Street in 1921. As the medical staff had mostly trained at St Peter's Hospital, the hospital increasingly focused on urology, with the venereal disease service being separated off. The hospital was renamed in 1927 as St Paul's Hospital for Diseases (including Cancer) of the Genito-Urinary Organs and Skin.

The start of the NHS in 1948 coincided with the availability of antibiotics, which promised to reduce venereal diseases from serious illnesses to a minor inconvenience. The need for specialist hospital care for venereal disease rapidly receded, leaving St Paul's and St Peter's, now combined and designated a postgraduate teaching hospital, to concentrate on urology. They were soon joined, in 1952, by St Philip's Hospital, which had been the Sheffield Street Hospital, run by London County Council for treating venereal disease, but was now broadening its remit to encompass other genito-urinary conditions. The position of St Paul's and St Peter's was enhanced in 1954 by the University of London establishing the Institute of Urology at St Peter's.

During the 1950s and 60s, the three hospitals coordinated their developments. In 1972, the Institute moved to the Shaftesbury Hospital (the former home of the Hôpital et Dispensaire Français), and in 1992 all four hospitals merged with the Middlesex Hospital and moved to Riding House Street. Finally, in 2005, urological services and the Institute moved to the new University College Hospital on Euston Road.

Walk 2: The lost hospitals of St Luke's

Highlights

- site of the world's first chest hospital (Royal Hospital for Diseases of the Chest)
- remains of one of London's largest workhouse infirmaries (Holborn & Finsbury Poor Law Union)
- former home of the leading hospital for bowel disease in the UK (St Mark's Hospital)
- site of the earliest voluntary hospital in London (French Huguenot Hospital)
- one of the leading ophthalmic hospitals in the world (Moorfields Eye Hospital)
- one of the last surviving public baths and washhouses in London
- site of one of the most spectacular buildings in 19th century London (St Luke's Hospital)

Start: Angel underground station
Finish: Old Street underground station
Length: 3.7 km (1.5 hours)

In 1733 the parish of St Luke's, less than a mile north of the City of London, was largely rural. Apart from the old City Pest House for plague victims, some almshouses, inns and tea gardens, this area was largely orchards, fields and moorland. But this was all soon to change. To the south, an expanding City hungry for land had drained Moorfields (modern-day Finsbury Circus to Finsbury Square) and laid out new streets and squares outside the City walls. This area was to become the centre of medical London up until 1800.

As the appetite for land grew, St Luke's was next in line. The rural tranquillity of the area was shattered in 1761 with the construction of City Road, which, for the first time, linked the City directly with Islington and beyond. This served to open up the area for development, a trend given further momentum when the Regent's Canal (with its City Road basin) was constructed in 1820. While such developments might have been expected to generate the manufacture and warehousing of goods, less predictable was its development as a centre for health care. Yet this is what happened. City Road was to witness the evolution of health care from the isolation and confinement of plague victims, through the establishment of workhouse infirmaries and voluntary hospitals, to the high-tech research establishments of the late 20th century.

This walk focuses largely on the extraordinary period up to 1900, by which time seven hospitals had been established in St Luke's. But almost as quickly, they were to vanish. Today, only one is still functioning.

And it was not just the hospitals that disappeared. The district of St Luke's itself became invisible. Although

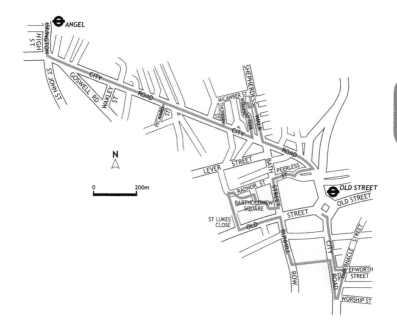

it still appears on street maps, few Londoners have heard of it, unlike the adjacent parishes of Finsbury, Clerkenwell, Hoxton and Shoreditch. This may have been the result of a deliberate policy to 'lose' one of the poorest, most deprived areas of London. Like St Giles (another parish that became invisible), much of the housing stock was dreadful, with overcrowded 'rookeries'. In the 1850s St Luke's had 245 people per acre, more than St Giles (221), Clerkenwell (170), Westminster (71) or Islington (30). The local Medical Officer of Health described the houses as 'typhus nests'. Both St Luke's and St Giles were 'dealt with' by wholesale redevelopment that left them almost unrecognisable, destroying as it did both the architectural heritage and any sense of community.

So why did this corner of rapidly expanding 19th century London play host to so many hospitals? There seem to be two reasons. First, the centre of 'medical London' in the 18th century was Moorfields. You were quite likely to encounter the leading doctors of the day as you strolled through Moorfields at that time, just as you might today in Marylebone. They were attracted there by the expanding merchant and business class from whom more money could be made than from the Court and aristocracy in the newly fashionable West End. Second, the area opened up by the construction of City Road offered the opportunity of relatively cheap land on which to build large institutions, an activity that was impossible in the City due to lack of space and the high cost of land.

And why were the hospitals lost? First, as with other areas of central London, the local population declined in number as people moved further out during the 19th and early 20th centuries, facilitated by improved public transport. Second, the 'healthy' rural environment that had initially proved so attractive to hospitals no longer existed. Third, as elsewhere, small specialist hospitals were not sustainable both for medical and for financial reasons. Fourth, along with many other buildings in St Luke's, considerable damage was inflicted in World War II by German bombing raids. And finally, the West End increasingly became a more attractive location for hospitals given the proximity of the new railway termini at Paddington, Euston, St Pancras and King's Cross bringing patients into London.

This walk gives you the opportunity to rediscover the lost hospitals of St Luke's. Their fortunes have been mixed: one is still functioning; one has survived though is no longer a hospital; parts of two still exist; but no trace remains of the other three. What all seven experienced was a never-ending struggle for funds, the challenge of balancing the power of doctors with that of governors, and the difficulty of recruiting and retaining well-trained nurses.

This walk also illustrates three other factors that have characterised health care for centuries. First is the influence of unlicensed practitioners on establishment medicine. Despite some reluctance on the part of formally educated and registered doctors to accept the contribution of others (often referred to as quacks, mountebanks or

charletans), the distinction is less clear than the medical profession would like. You will see how an itinerant oculist established the specialty of ophthalmology, how clerics and other 18th century 'empirics' adopted and developed electrotherapy, which was, in time, to become a key element in the treatment of mental illness and of paralysis, and how proponents of Turkish baths influenced rheumatology.

Second, despite all the complex biomedical developments over the past hundred years, water has played several remarkable roles in promoting health and treating disease. Apart from the provision of clean drinking water from free public fountains and the establishment of public baths and washhouses to improve hygiene, water was used as therapy for musculoskeletal conditions (Turkish and other specialist baths) and for treating insanity (by the shock induced by cold water plunges).

And finally, the walk illustrates one feature of the more recent past, the contribution of lay organisations representing the needs and interests of particular groups of patients. While some organisations have remained quite small and local, others have become significant players in national policy-making. Largely funded by charity, they campaign, lobby policy-makers, fund research, educate and inform both the public and professionals, and provide support and services for patients and their carers. On the walk you will see the national headquarters of three such organisations.

Our walk starts at the Angel underground station. On leaving the station, turn left along Islington High Street and at the traffic lights turn left into City Road. Stop after about 50 m outside the national headquarters of the National Autistic Society.

Until the 18th century, the only road connecting Islington with the City of London was St John's Street (running south via Smithfield to Newgate). Otherwise, only country lanes ran east and west from the Angel. All this changed in 1756 with the construction of the New Road (present-day Pentonville Road), which ran west to Battlebridge (King's Cross) and beyond to Paddington, and in 1761 when City Road connected Islington to the City via the parish of St Luke's. These two roads were, in effect, a bypass for traffic to travel east–west without having to go via the increasingly congested West End.

You are standing outside the headquarters of the **National Autistic Society**, one of the largest of thousands of lay organisations in the UK that represent the interests of patients and their carers. It was established in 1962 by a group of parents frustrated at the lack of understanding, service provision and support for their autistic children. Like other national lay organisations, it has a huge membership (13,000), regional offices, an elected council and a chief executive. It champions the rights and interests of those who are autistic, campaigns for better statutory services, and provides services and training.

Walk on for about 200 m, cross over to the other (south) side of City Road, and after another 200 m

stop outside the former **St Mark's Hospital**, recently converted to upmarket apartments that have retained the name, St Mark's. This is an example of the numerous voluntary specialist hospitals (p. 119) created in London between 1750 and 1900. Like the four others you will encounter on this walk, St Mark's started life in the City and moved to City Road when it had outgrown its original facilities. This area offered a greenfield site with few restrictions on space and considerably cheaper land than in the City.

As with other specialist hospitals, the instigator, Frederick Salmon, was an ambitious surgeon whose progress and advancement were obstructed by medical nepotism and corruption. In 1835 he opened the Benevolent Dispensary for the Relief of the Poor Afflicted with Fistula, Piles and Other Diseases of the Rectum in Aldersgate Street, referred to at the time as the 'Fistula Infirmary'. Many of his subscribers had themselves suffered from lower bowel problems (a common problem at the time given people's diet) and had cause to be grateful for Salmon's help. They included William Copeland (Lord Mayor of London), Charles Dickens (who suffered from anal fistula) and Lord Iveagh (of the Guinness brewing empire).

By 1838 the infirmary needed more space. It first moved to Charterhouse Square and then in 1853 to a fine new, three-storey, Italianate building designed by John Wallen (the right-hand side of the building you see today). It had 25 beds for inpatients together with outpatient facilities. One to benefit

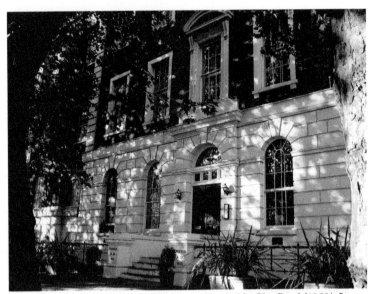

The main entrance to the original St Mark's Hospital in City Road (1853). It expanded several times (part of the 1926 extension can be seen on the left) before moving to Harrow in 1995

was the artist Walter Sickert, whose treatment at St Mark's has been used as evidence that he suffered from an anal fistula and not, as those who believe he was Jack the Ripper have alleged, a penile fistula (which would have rendered him impotent and therefore, they claim, more likely to be a serial killer of women).

Significantly, in 1854 the infirmary acquired a new name – St Mark's Hospital for Fistula and other Diseases of the Rectum. It was common practice among specialist hospitals to pick a saint's name so as to make fund-raising easier. However, Salmon was insistent that the public should know what went on in the new building by inscribing in the stonework across the front of the building 'St Mark's Hospital for Fistula &c'. (The lettering

has been covered by the developers, perhaps fearing it might put off potential residents.)

In 1896 the hospital expanded to the rear of the original building. (This can be seen if you look in through the gates of the car park to the right of the building.) Although there were now 54 beds, financial constraints meant that only half could be used. Fund-raising events – dinners, balls, theatre performances (including one organised by Lillie Langtry) – contributed to solving the problem. The increasing importance of bowel cancer led to another change of name in 1909 to St Mark's Hospital for Cancer, Fistula &c. Staff here played a leading role in establishing the British Empire Cancer Campaign (a precursor of the present-day Cancer Research UK).

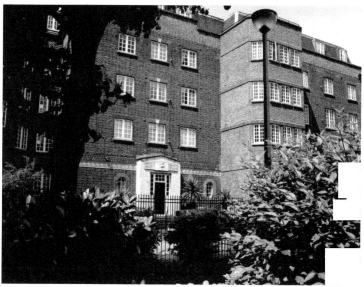

St Mark's Hospital Nurses' Home (1926), with a bas-relief of a winged lion, the symbol of St Mark, over the door. Like the adjoining hospital, it was converted to private apartments in the 1990s

During World War I, the hospital purchased the neighbouring Congregational Chapel, and in 1926 built the wing that constitutes the left-hand side of the building. It also built a nurses' home (p. 151) to help attract and retain nurses, which can be seen if you walk about 50 m down Pickard Street, along the left side of the hospital. You can see the original entrance to the nurses' home surmounted by a bas-relief of a winged lion, the symbol of St Mark. In 1948 the hospital, which Aneurin Bevan called 'a jewel in his health service', became part of the NHS, and in 1995 it moved to Harrow to be amalgamated with Northwick Park Hospital, where it continues to be the national centre for large bowel diseases.

Return to City Road where, on the opposite side at No. 275, was **Smith's Baths**, one of many privately run baths and washhouses that were established in the second half of the 19th century. As you continue along City Road, immediately on your right is Kestrel House, which was the site of No. 266, where the **Municipal Throat & Ear Infirmary** was established in 1877. It was one of seven ENT hospitals (p. 82) in London in the late 19th century, surviving until 1927.

The importance of making water (p. 259) publicly available, given the inadequate or non-existent supply in many people's homes, can be seen a few metres further on, having crossed Central Street, where there is one of the original granite cattle troughs installed by the **Metropolitan Water Fountain & Cattle Trough Association**. The lack of clean drinking water and the high level of alcohol consumption (partly a consequence of the former) in 19th century London were of increasing concern to public health advocates, the Church and the temperance movement. The Association was established in 1859 by Samuel Gurney, an MP and philanthropist, and Edward Wakefield, a barrister. Originally called the Metropolitan Free Drinking Fountain Association, it expanded to include 'cattle' troughs in 1867, although these were actually for horses, the principal means of transport for both people and goods. Sites of fountains and troughs were the petrol stations of their day, creating a focus for people to gather and converse.

Cross back over to the north side of City Road and continue, passing the City Road canal basin on your left. In the 19th century, a Patent Capsule Manufactory (for making proprietary medicines) occupied the site that is now occupied by a petrol station. Turn left immediately after the petrol station and stop after 10 m where you will see on the right **Thoresby House**, a five-storey, Italianate yellow and red-brick building. It was built as a nurses' home in 1905 for the Royal Hospital for Diseases of the Chest, which stood behind it, facing City Road. All that remains of the hospital is a tiny remnant of the wall that enclosed its grounds, which can be seen beside the pavement, to the right of the nurses' home. After the closure of the hospital, Thoresby House continued as a nurses' home for two other local hospitals before becoming a hall of residence for American students studying in London.

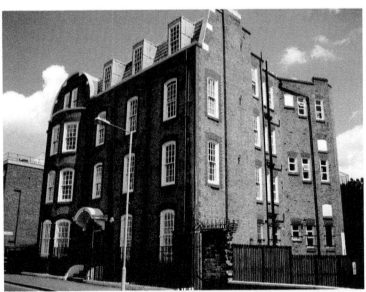

The nurses' home for the Royal Hospital for Diseases of the Chest, built in 1905. All that remains of the hospital, a tiny remnant of the girdling wall, can be seen in the foreground

The Royal Hospital for Diseases of the Chest was the first specialist hospital, not just in Britain but in the world, for diseases of the chest, particularly tuberculosis (p. 218). It was founded in 1814 by a doctor, Isaac Buxton, and like St Mark's Hospital, it started life in the City. It moved here in 1849 because the site offered fresh air and was not hemmed in by neighbouring buildings. Following several extensions during the rest of the century, it achieved a capacity of 80 beds. On average, patients stayed for five weeks.

In 1921 the hospital was amalgamated with the Great Northern Hospital in Holloway. Inpatient facilities had to be moved there following bomb damage in 1941, but the outpatient service continued here. In 1948 both hospitals were incorporated into the NHS, and soon after the remaining services here were moved to Holloway, the building being demolished in the 1950s. The only reminder of the past glory of this site is the block of flats, Buxton Court, named after the hospital's founder.

Return to City Road. On the other (south) side of City Road at No. 238 you can see the national headquarters of one of the oldest and largest lay organisations in the country, **The Stroke Association**. This started life in 1898 with a quite different concern – tuberculosis. The National Association for the Prevention of Consumption was established to educate the public and treat patients. With the demise of TB and increasing concern about heart disease in the middle of the

Walk 2

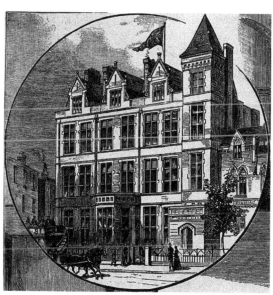

The new wing for the Royal Hospital for Diseases of the Chest (1885) attached to the original 1849 building, part of which can be seen on the right. The hospital moved in 1950 and these buildings were demolished

20th century, it became The Chest & Heart Association. Then in 1992 its focus shifted again, this time onto stroke. An idea of the scale of its activities can be gained from the 170 community projects it runs nationwide.

Continue along the north side of City Road to Wellesley Terrace, which forms the eastern boundary of the old St Luke's Workhouse. Cross Wellesley Terrace and look through the gates at the extensive site, now largely abandoned and used as a car park.

Workhouse infirmaries

From 1601 responsibility for paupers lay with the 15,000 parishes that, from local rates, provided 'outdoor relief' (similar to social security benefits) and workhouses. Most of the latter included a rudimentary infirmary to house the sick and infirm. Concern about the cost of outdoor relief led to the 1834 Poor Law Amendment Act, which discouraged it. If people wanted help, they had to succumb to the misery of the workhouse.

The Act also shifted responsibility from individual parishes to 573 Unions covering larger areas. Each of the 17 Unions created in London (and five London parishes that retained their responsibilities) was controlled by a Board of Guardians, usually local tradesmen or shopkeepers. Between 1834 and 1839 many new workhouses were built that included infirmaries, although space per person was half that designated for prisons. In exceptional circumstances, the Guardians would pay for an inmate to be transferred to a voluntary hospital for treatment.

Infirmaries struggled to compete with voluntary hospitals and private practice for staff. The cost of medications had to be met by the poorly paid medical officer, thus creating a financial disincentive to treat.

In 1866, 21,000 patients in London were being cared for by only 142 trained nurses, with most care carried out by untrained inmates (pauper nurses). Despite these difficulties, workhouse infirmaries were treating more patients than the voluntary hospitals. The patients were more likely to be medical than surgical, to suffer from chronic conditions and to be older.

Two Inquiries confirmed the scale of the deficiencies. In addition, there was acceptance of the need to plan services for infectious diseases. The Metropolitan Asylums Board (p. 179) was established, which provided the first opportunity for a London-wide planning of health services. Among other measures, it was required to provide hospitals for the poor under the control of a doctor, rather than a workhouse master, and to establish Poor Law Dispensaries. Finance came from central funds such that the richer districts subsidised the poorer ones. The Board merged the Unions and parishes into six Sick Asylum Districts and required them to establish hospitals on sites separate from workhouses. Due to the higher than anticipated costs, only two Districts ever built new premises; the other four simply upgraded existing facilities.

Workhouse infirmaries continued to differ from voluntary general hospitals (p. 148) in several ways: they seldom admitted accident or emergency cases; had no attached medical school; had no post-mortem facilities; and there was no restriction on the types of patient admitted. In addition, it was not until 1873 that people could be treated as outpatients when Poor Law Dispensaries were established (despite having existed in Ireland for 25 years). By 1890 there were 44 in London.

By then, the need for workhouses was declining as a result of new services being introduced: lunatic asylums, epileptic colonies and mental subnormality asylums. And during the early 20th century, further measures reduced needs further: old-age pensions, children's homes, National Insurance, venereal disease services and TB sanatoria. The workhouse infirmaries became public (municipal) hospitals, complementing the voluntary hospitals, and both were incorporated into the NHS.

When St Luke's parish became part of the Holborn & Finsbury Poor Law Union in 1869, this served as the workhouse infirmary (p. 54) for the Union, with able-bodied inmates being housed in their other workhouse in Gray's Inn Road. In recognition of the new role, a trained nurse, Louisa Mullucks, was employed. To care for 105 patients (including 42 fever cases), she was supported by three pauper nurses, two of whom were in their late 60s. A Commission, established by medical journal *The Lancet*, was in no doubt about the limitations of pauper nurses:

'The majority of them are aged and feeble and past work, or have strong tendencies to drink, and in many cases have otherwise led vicious lives … in the great majority of cases, pauper nurses can only manage their patients by inspiring fear, and that their conduct is consequently often brutal.'

Despite criticisms from social reformers, the infirmary expanded, and in 1916, when it was renamed the Holborn & Finsbury Institution, it accommodated over 1,100 patients. In 1936, in an attempt to distance it further from its workhouse origins, it was renamed again as **St Matthew's Hospital** (after the local church on City Road). During World War II, it suffered bomb damage, during which 83 patients and three nurses were killed. As a result, it closed for the rest of the war. It became part of the NHS in 1948 and was modernised in the 1960s, being used as a geriatric hospital until 1987 when it closed. Although most of the hospital was demolished, some of the 19th century buildings remain, as does this entrance to the site, complete with the initials 'SM' on the gates.

Walk up Wellesley Terrace, along the outside of the original perimeter wall. Note the 1832 parish boundary

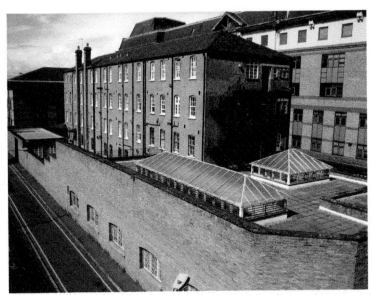

The four-storey ward block for female 'imbeciles' built in the 1860s is all that remains of St Luke's Workhouse Infirmary, apart from the girdling wall that can be seen in the foreground

marker, set in the wall (where the wall changes direction), showing that half the workhouse site was not actually located within the parish of St Luke. Near the end of Wellesley Terrace, turn right through a pair of gates and enter the site. Just inside, you will see the only remaining hospital building, the old ward block for 'imbeciles', converted in the 1950s to a nurses' home (now called Ashwell House), and in the courtyard the remains of some of the outbuildings.

Walk down the steps in front of you and round the north end of Ashwell House. You can leave the site through an archway under the modern office block ahead of you onto Shepherdess Walk. (If this way is closed, you will need to return to Wellesley Street,

turn right and then right along Micawber Street and at the end, right into Shepherdess Walk.) Turn right and head back down to City Road. On the left-hand side used to stand **Lady Lumley's Almshouses**, built at a time when the area was fields and orchards. Part of the original perimeter wall and fence of the workhouse infirmary can be seen on the right as you approach City Road. The brick pillars carry the initials 'HU' for the Holborn (& Finsbury Poor Law) Union.

Just before reaching City Road, you will see the Eagle Tavern on the left, built on the site of the Shepherd & Shepherdess Inn, an alehouse and tea garden established in 1743. The gardens provided an escape for city residents, particularly the infirm, seeking fresh air. Invalids sometimes stayed at the inn:

> 'To the Shepherd and
> Shepherdess then they go,
>
> To tea with their wives, for a
> constant rule;
>
> And next cross the road to the
> Fountain also,
>
> And there they all sit, so
> pleasant and cool,
>
> And see, in and out,
>
> The folk walk about,
>
> And the gentlemen angling in
> Peerless Pool.'

As you will see in a moment, The Fountain pub survives in Peerless Street on the other side of City Road.

Stop when you reach City Road. From this spot, in 1865, you could have seen six hospitals, all of which have disappeared. Looking back up City Road, you would have seen St Mark's and the Royal Hospital for Diseases of the Chest. Close by was St Luke's Workhouse Infirmary. Down the road that joins City Road on the other side, the French Huguenot Hospital and St Luke's Hospital for Lunatics would have been visible. And, to your left, at the end of City Road, the City of London Lying-In Hospital. To see the only functioning hospital here today, the Royal London Ophthalmic Hospital, cross City Road at the pelican crossing, turn left and walk 200 m until you reach Cayton Street and the new main entrance to the hospital. It is in the King George V extension, built in the 1930s and funded by a public appeal. Above the

door is a fine sculpture by Eric Gill of the restoration of sight to blind Bartimaeus. Continue along City Road for 40 m to the main entrance of the original building.

In 1805, John Cunningham Saunders founded the London Dispensary for Curing Diseases of the Eye and Ear in Charterhouse Square, only the second eye hospital (p. 59) to be established in London. The first had been set up just three months earlier by an oculist, Jonathan Wathen, who had no formal medical training or qualification. Increasing demand led Saunders to expand by moving to a new purpose-built home in 1822 in Lower Moorfields (Finsbury Circus). Its success was marked by its being redesignated the Royal London Ophthalmic Hospital in 1837.

By the late 19th century, the building was proving increasingly inadequate. An additional challenge was the change going on around the hospital: construction of the London & North-Western Railway's goods station, Broad Street station and Liverpool Street station made the area noisy and disturbing. The final straw was the need for street widening. Given the high value of the site plus the need to expand, the hospital governors opted to move further out from the centre of London and rebuild on cheaper land here in City Road.

The red-brick building you see today was completed in 1898 and opened in 1899. The main entrance was felt to be too grand for use by the patients, who had to enter via a side door. Financial constraints meant that only 70 of the 138 beds could initially be used, and even by

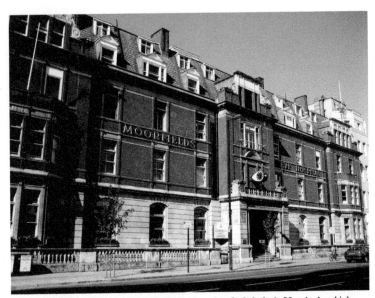

The third and current home for the Royal London Ophthalmic Hospital, which opened in City Road in 1899. Patients had to use a side door as the main entrance was considered too grand

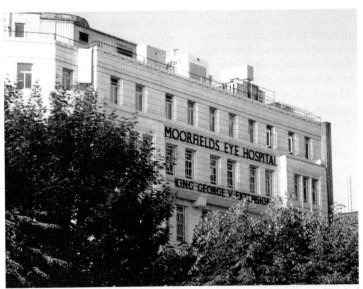

The King George V Extension was added to the Royal London Ophthalmic Hospital in 1935, and the hospital was renamed Moorfields Eye Hospital in 1956

Eye hospitals

Until 1800 eye disease was mainly in the hands of unlicensed oculists. The only specialist hospital to have been established, St John's Hospital for Diseases of the Eyes, Legs & Breasts, in Holborn in 1771, survived only two years. The situation changed with the spread of a serious eye infection in Britain following the return, in 1803, of British troops from campaigns against Napoleon in Egypt. Three voluntary specialist hospitals (p. 119) were established: in 1804, Jonathan Wathen, an oculist, opened the Royal Infirmary for Diseases of the Eye in Cork Street; a year later, John Cunningham Saunders established the London Dispensary for Curing Diseases of the Eye and Ear in Charterhouse Square, which, from 1808, concentrated on eyes as the London Infirmary for Curing Diseases of the Eye; and in 1816 the Infirmary for Diseases of the Eye was established by George Guthrie in St Giles.

To meet the growing demand, two of the hospitals expanded: in 1822, the London Infirmary moved to a new building in Lower Moorfields (Finsbury Circus) and became the Royal London Ophthalmic Hospital in 1837; and Guthrie's Infirmary moved to new premises in Covent Garden in 1844 and, in 1854, was renamed the Royal Westminster Ophthalmic Hospital. In addition, three new hospitals were founded: the Central London Ophthalmic Hospital (1843) near Brunswick Square, which moved to Gray's Inn Road in 1848; the Western Ophthalmic Hospital (1856) in Paddington; and the Royal Eye Hospital (1857).

Ophthalmology advanced following the introduction in the 1850s of the ophthalmoscope, which allowed doctors to look inside the eye. As general hospitals started establishing eye departments, the first of several mergers of specialist hospitals took place when, in 1872, the Royal London Ophthalmic Hospital acquired the assets of the Cork Street infirmary. This, together with other factors, necessitated a move, in 1899, to City Road. Meanwhile, the Central London had long outlived its house in Gray's Inn Road and suggested joining the Royal London in City Road. The latter, however, 'entertained no idea of amalgamation', so instead the Central London built a new home in Judd Street, although it did not move there until 1925. A year later, the Royal Westminster left its Charing Cross home and moved to Holborn.

World War II was to be the trigger that led to mergers. Bomb damage at City Road necessitated the transfer of the Royal London outpatient department to the Central London building in Judd Street. After the war, a merger finally took place between the three principal eye hospitals in north and east London, creating the Moorfields, Westminster and Central Eye Hospital. By concentrating clinical services at City Road and Holborn, the University of London was able to establish its Institute of Ophthalmology in the Judd Street building. In recognition of both its 19th century location and common usage, the merged institution was officially renamed Moorfields Eye Hospital in 1956. The merger was completed when the Holborn branch closed, and in 1988 the Institute of Ophthalmology moved to custom-built premises at City Road.

1913 only 118 were in use. However, the spare capacity was put to good use as accommodation for nurses.

In the early years of World War II, the hospital was fortunate to escape with only minor damage from bombing raids. The need to devote all available hospitals in London to trauma and surgical emergencies led to eye patients being evacuated. The hospital's luck ran out on 29 July 1944 when a flying bomb struck and caused such extensive damage that it was proposed to pull the hospital down and relocate to a greenfield site. Instead, following the war, it was decided to merge the three leading eye hospitals in central London to create Moorfields, Westminster and Central Eye Hospital, shortened in 1956 to Moorfields Eye Hospital. Although it then took 40 years to achieve, the three hospitals plus the University of London's Institute of Ophthalmology were eventually brought together on this site in 1988.

Continue along City Road and turn right into Peerless Street. After 150 m stop outside the new Children's Eye Centre. The street name and the Old Fountain pub you have just passed, mentioned in the 18th century poem above, are reminders of the area's past. Standing here in 1880 you would have seen the **Peerless Pool** stretching away to the south (now St Luke's Estate) and, beyond it, the back of St Luke's Hospital for Lunatics (which you will learn more about in a while). In the 17th century, springs in this area overflowed and created what, in 1603, Stowe described as: 'cleare

water called the Perilous Pond because divers youths by swimming therein have been drowned'. In 1743 Mr William Kemp, an eminent jeweller who claimed to have derived relief from violent headaches by bathing in the water, created:

> *'the completest swimming*
> *bath in the whole world …*
> *He [Kemp] spared no expense*
> *nor contrivances to render it*
> *quite private and retired from*
> *public inspection, decent in its*
> *regulations and as genteel in its*
> *furniture as such a place could be.'*

Designed by John Cleghorn, it was on a grand scale – 170 feet long, 108 feet wide and 3–5 feet deep, and entered through a marble pavilion. It was surrounded by compartments for changing outside which were lofty banks covered with shrubs and a terraced walk planted with lime trees. Four pairs of marble steps descended to the bath, which had a fine gravel bottom. There was also a covered cold bath (36 feet by 18 feet), supplied with water from a particularly cold spring, faced with marble and paved with stone. In addition, between where you are standing and the end of Peerless Street ahead, was a huge fish pond, beyond which stood the French Huguenot Hospital (see below). The Peerless Pool survived until 1869, when it was filled in and built over. Its existence has not, however, been entirely forgotten. A crime novel, set in 1758 and based on the detective work of an apothecary, *Death in the Peerless Pool* by Deryn Lake, was published in 1999.

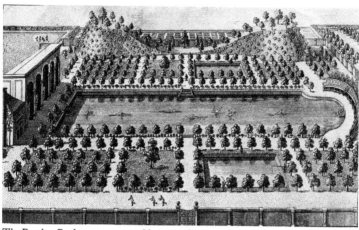

The Peerless Pool was constructed in 1743 for 'Gentlemen Lovers of Swimming & Bathing', although the owner claimed there were also health benefits. It survived until 1869

Continue straight on along Peerless Street and stop when you reach Bath Street. On your right is the modern home of one of the University of London's postgraduate institutes (p. 101), the Institute of Ophthalmology, opened in 1992. Bath Street was originally known as Pest House Lane but was renamed to avoid harming the image of the Peerless Pool. The land on the other side of Bath Street and slightly to the left was the site of the **City Pest House** in the 17th century.

The rapid growth of urban populations in the late medieval period, combined with the need to contain people within the town or city walls, led to increasing overcrowding. Despite attempts to stop the spread of infectious diseases through measures such as imposing quarantine on travellers, infections repeatedly spread across Europe. Like other cities, London established a pest house outside the city walls for isolating people thought to have or to be incubating an infection, in particular plague. They were often positioned on the edge of a churchyard for ease of burial, not the most encouraging sight for those confined to the Pest House.

There was considerable resistance on the part of both patients and staff to being confined to such buildings. The high mortality suffered by staff led some to suggest that patients should be 'cured at a distance' by having them shout out their symptoms and, in reply, an apothecary would shout out the treatment. The pest house established here in 1593, beside a plague pit (for the burial of victims), was paid for by proceeds from the Spanish Armada. At that time, it was over half a mile from the city. Despite appearances (in a contemporary print), it could accommodate 200–300 people.

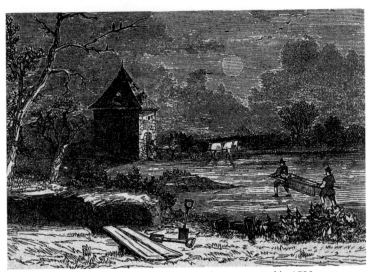

The City Pest House for plague victims was, when constructed in 1593, some distance from the city. From 1693 to 1717 it was used as a hospital by French Huguenot refugees, before being demolished

By the end of the 17th century, the threat of plague was receding and the pest house fell into disuse. However, another use for the building was about to arise. The Revocation of the Edict of Nantes in 1685 left Huguenots (French protestants) feeling vulnerable. Many fled to England (many settling in Shoreditch and Spitalfields), where they found none of the hospital care they were familiar with in France. In desperation, they took over the abandoned pest house in 1693 and used it to care for sick members of their growing community, an example of the specific provision of health care for foreigners (p. 19).

In 1708 Jacques de Gastigny left £1,000 in his Will to be of benefit to the refugees he had seen in pitiable conditions at the Pest House. The Huguenots were familiar with the French approach to creating and maintaining hospitals through donations from better-off citizens. The establishment of the **French Huguenot Hospital** (known as La Providence) set an example of what could be achieved by the voluntary actions of concerned citizens. While St Bartholomew's, St Thomas' and St Mary of Bethlehem (Bethlem) Hospitals depended on endowments, the French Huguenot Hospital was the first voluntary hospital (dependent on subscribers) to be established in Britain. Within a decade, several other voluntary general hospitals were being planned.

The new hospital, designed by Jacob Gibbs, was built in 1718 on land adjoining the Pest House (now the site of St Luke's Primary School). It accommodated 80 people in three buildings in a plain Georgian style, set around a

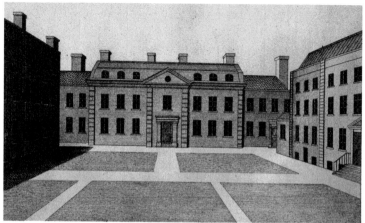

French Huguenot Hospital (1718), designed by Jacob Gibbs, was the first voluntary hospital in London. Although the hospital moved in 1865, the building survived until the 1960s

quadrangle and facing north (onto present-day Radnor Street). With the addition of more buildings in 1760, it could accommodate 234. The hospital cared for all types of patient including 'distracted persons' (mentally ill) such as poor Jacques Ray, a goldsmith, who took to 'running about the streets like a madman, forsaking his business and crying Oranges and Lemons'.

By the start of the 19th century, the hospital was in decline. The city had spread, the rural surroundings were gone, and the Huguenots themselves had become absorbed into English society. Despite this, the hospital continued until 1865, when it moved to Hackney and subsequently, in 1960, changed its role to that of an almshouse and moved to Rochester, Kent. The building here survived until the 1960s, when it was demolished as part of widespread clearances.

Turn left and walk along Bath Street. Despite the presence of the pest house, the rural tranquillity of the area in the 16th and 17th centuries made it a favoured location for almshouses. On the left were **Alleyn's Almshouses**, built in 1620 to house three men and seven women, then rebuilt in 1707 and again in 1874. Residents received a pension of 6 pence a week and a new cloak or gown every two years. A nurse from the Finsbury Dispensary (near The Angel) met their health care needs. The almshouses survived until the 1960s when they too were demolished, to make way for the high-rise flats that you see today.

At the end of the modern two-storey car park on the right-hand side of Bath Street, you will see a plaque on the wall commemorating the City Pest House. To the left of the plaque, Leage Street used to run

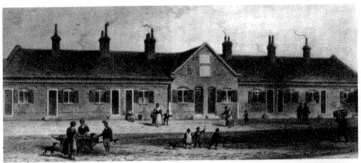

Alleyn's Almshouses (1707) had been established in 1620 by actor–manager Edward Alleyn. Rebuilt again in 1874, they were demolished in the clearances of the 1960s

from where you are standing through to St Luke's church, the spire of which can be seen. Walk towards it, entering Steadman Court. Turn right towards Cope House where, on the left, you can exit to Lizard Street. Walk to the right along Lizard Street, and after about 20 m turn left into a small park, Radnor Street Gardens. Exit at the far end onto Radnor Street, turn left and stop at the junction with Ironmonger Row.

To your right is **Finsbury Borough Council Public Baths & Washhouse**, an example of municipal recognition of the importance of water to health. In 1846 the Baths and Washhouse Act empowered local authorities to provide swimming baths, washhouses and slipper baths. Despite believing that baths would improve not only people's health but also their morals, these baths were not built until 1931. Before then, if they could afford it, the poor of St Luke's would have to travel to one of the private baths such as Smith's, which you saw on City Road.

Unlike most public baths, the two-storey building faced in stone in the Roman revival style with patterned glazing to the upper windows, a cornice and a pantiled roof is still functioning today. The health benefits of baths were not seen as being limited to personal hygiene. In the late 19th century, increasing interest among the medical profession in the health benefits of Turkish baths led to over 100 being established in London. The baths here include three hot rooms, a vapour room and cold plunge pools.

Turn left and walk down the pedestrianised Ironmonger Row, past St Luke's church (designed by Nicholas Hawksmoor and John James) to Old Street. Like other churches, St Luke's, from 1882 until 1950, ran a Sick Benefit Society, a social insurance scheme in which the working poor contributed a small weekly payment to fund their use of health care.

Turn left into Old Street and walk along to the junction with Bath Street. Cross Old Street and walk 50 m

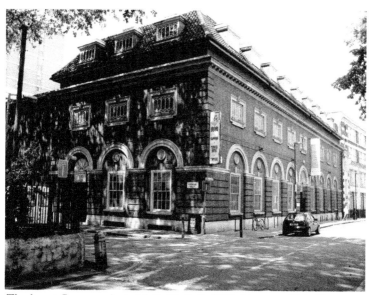

The elegant, Roman revival-style Public Baths & Washhouse established by Finsbury Borough Council in 1931 is one of few such establishments still functioning

down Bunhill Row, stopping opposite Featherstone Street. In 1740 a barber-surgeon, John Harrison, established the London Infirmary in a house on the right-hand side of the street (long since demolished). He employed a Huguenot refugee, John Andree from Rheims, as physician, but within six months its 30 beds proved inadequate and he relocated to Aldgate. It was eventually to become one of the largest and most prestigious hospitals in the city, the Royal London Hospital at Whitechapel. The site here is now the headquarters of another national patient organisation, Action on Hearing Loss (previously the Royal National Institute for Deaf People).

Continue for another 100 m and turn left to walk through Bunhill Fields Burial Ground. The site of burials since Saxon times, it probably acquired the name Bone Hill in the 16th century when about 1,000 cartloads of human bones were dumped here, removed from St Paul's Cathedral charnel-house to make room for new interments. From 1661 until 1885, 120,000 religious dissenters were buried here, including Blake, Bunyan and Defoe.

On leaving the Burial Fields, cross City Road and walk 150 m to the right to the junction with Tabernacle Street and Worship Street. In 1750, partly in response to the Royal Bethlehem Hospital (as St Mary of Bethlehem Hospital had become, having moved to beside the city wall, 400 m south of here) being unable to meet demand, and partly

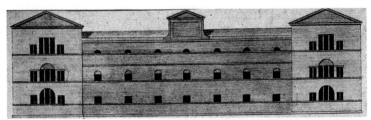

The original St Luke's Hospital for Lunatics, designed by George Dance the Elder in 1750, was used only until 1786, when it moved to new premises designed by George Dance's son

through concern about the perceived abuses that lunatics suffered in that hospital, a group decided to establish an alternative hospital for the care and treatment of 'lunatics' (defined as those with mental illness (p. 66) that was deemed curable). The site identified was that now occupied by the first few buildings along the left-hand side of Worship Street. George Dance the Elder designed **St Luke's Hospital for Lunatics**, a 'neat but very plain edifice … a building of considerable length, plastered over and whitened, with ranges of small square windows on which no decorations have been bestowed'.

The first chief physician was Dr William Battie. Renowned as 'an eccentric humorist', he shared the founders' view that 'the patients of this hospital shall not be exposed to publick view'. Consistent with the medical thinking of the day, there was a large cold plunge bath to shake lunatics out of their insanity. Although a system of non-restraint was professed, manacles and other restraints were sometimes used. By 1786 the hospital needed to expand, and a new site was found about 400 m north of here, which you will see in a few minutes.

Walk up the left side of Tabernacle Street and stop opposite

Mental illness

Just as religion had been the dominant concern in society in the 17th century, insanity was in the 18th century. Up until 1700 the only public institution for 'lunatics' was St Mary of Bethlehem Hospital. Founded in 1377 it was one of five 'royal' hospitals to be re-endowed by the Crown and administered by the Corporation of London following the Reformation in the 1530s. Known

as Bethlem or Bedlam, it was rebuilt in 1675, just outside the City walls in Moorfields (Finsbury Circus), to accommodate 130 patients.

The perceived need to confine 'lunatics' led, from 1670, to the establishment of private madhouses, particularly in Hoxton and Clerkenwell. They varied in size from 'single houses' for confining the affluent (including royalty, such as George III in 1788) to institutions housing several hundred. Concern about both the conditions in many of them, and the fact that people (mostly women) who were quite sane were frequently confined because male relatives wanted them out of the way, led to the Madhouse Act in 1774, which established inspections by Royal College of Physicians commissioners. Inspection was strengthened after a second Act in 1828, which allowed inspectors to release people and to revoke licences. By then, there were 48 madhouses in London.

Meanwhile, public provision was limited to Bethlem, workhouses, a lunatic ward at Guy's Hospital from 1723 and St Luke's Hospital, established in Moorfields (Finsbury Square) in 1751. In 1808 the County Asylums Act permitted local authorities to levy a rate to build asylums, but by 1844 only 15 had been built in England. So a second Act (1845) was passed that 'required' their construction, a responsibility in London taken over by the Metropolitan Asylums Board (p. 179) in 1867. Between 1831 and 1893 seven huge asylums were constructed on the outskirts of London.

At first this development was driven by a spirit of optimism that patients could be cured, but from about 1860 this gave way to pessimism. Instead, the asylums, with an average of 1,200 patients each, became places of containment and exclusion. It was not until 1923, and the establishment of the first mental hospital in London (the Maudsley) by the London County Council, that attempts at treating mental illness commenced.

The incorporation of all public hospitals and asylums into the NHS in 1948 coincided with a change in policy. For several reasons, the emphasis was to switch from large isolated institutions to incorporating the mentally ill in local general hospitals during their acute illnesses and caring for them in the community with domiciliary services. By the 1980s the 19th century asylums were being closed and sold to private developers for housing. Meanwhile, from the 1890s the private madhouses had been closing such that there were only eight left in London by 1959 when the Mental Health Act redesignated them as mental nursing homes.

Bonhill Street. The left side of Bonhill Street, opposite the back of the old St Luke's Hospital, had been the site of a cannon foundry until 1716, when it was seriously damaged by an explosion. It lay unused until 1739, when John Wesley, the Anglican clergyman who founded Methodism (so-called because of the members' methodical Christian life) bought the lease, repaired the building and used it as a chapel and his London headquarters for the next 40 years. Along with the chapel, he established a schoolroom and a **dispensary** for treating the poor.

John Wesley believed that he had to offer his congregation not only a better form of Christianity, but also a better form of medicine. In the 18th century, it was not uncommon

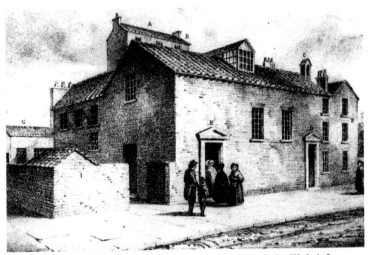

The old cannon foundry in Tabernacle Street that served as John Wesley's first headquarters for Methodism from 1739 to 1778 and included a dispensary for the poor

for clerics, especially in rural areas, to prescribe and dispense simple medical remedies to their needy parishioners. Wesley thought that 'regular physicians do exceedingly little good' compared with the 'empirics' who were commonly dismissed as quacks and charlatans.

In 1747 he made his own contribution to empowering lay people when he published *Primitive Physick, or an essay and natural way of curing most diseases*, primarily aimed at the poor who could not afford expensive remedies. It dealt with 288 conditions that he believed could be prevented or cured with herbs, water-drinking or cold bathing. His belief in the benefits of water extended, it is reported, to him plunging into the Thames to stop a violent nosebleed.

By 1760 he had become a leading practitioner and advocate of another form of therapy, electricity (p. 69), which he viewed as a cheap and effective means of treating the poor who attended his dispensary. He became one of the most notable electrotherapists in the 18th century. The impact on established medicine was quite rapid. In 1763 the Middlesex Hospital purchased a machine, and by the 1780s electrotherapy had become the stock in trade of many physicians. While most of the uses were later to be abandoned, electrotherapy found a role in psychiatry and in the treatment of paralysis. The Foundry was abandoned in 1778, when a new chapel was built, which you will now visit.

Continue along Tabernacle Street, turn left into Epworth

Electricity

Although William Gilbert had described magnetism in his work, *De Magnette*, in 1600, the first book in English on the subject, *The Subtil Medium Prov'd* by Richard Lovett, did not appear until 1756. Lovett was a clerk who, inspired by an itinerant lecturer, had started electrotherapeutic experiments in 1749. The involuntary twitching of muscles resulting from electric shocks gave hope that paralysis could be cured. There were three ways in which electricity was used: the electric bath in which the patient was electrified while insulated on a cake of resin or glass supports; the drawing of sparks from the body; and the administration of light shocks through a part of the body. The list of conditions that it was claimed could be successfully treated by electricity grew steadily over the following few decades to include renal stones, sciatica, pleurisy, stomach ache, ague, toothache, wens, deafness, gout and impotence.

John Wesley, the founder of Methodism, viewed electricity as a cheap and effective means of treating the poor who attended his dispensary in Moorfields. In 1756 he acquired his own machine and gradually increased the time he devoted to using it. He recorded his experiences in *The Desideratum: or, Electricity made plain and useful by a lover of mankind, and of Common Sense*, published, anonymously, in 1760. He became one of the most notable electrotherapists in the 18th century. Another practitioner was Jean-Paul Marat, a Swiss physician who came to London in 1765 and set up an electrotherapeutic practice in the West End, where he remained for 12 years before returning to France to be a key figure in the revolution of 1789.

The impact on establishment medicine was quite rapid. The Middlesex Hospital purchased a machine in 1765, St Bartholomew's Hospital did so in 1777, and St Thomas' Hospital created an electrical department. By the 1780s electrotherapy had become the stock in trade of many physicians who claimed that static electricity was helpful in the treatment of chorea (involuntary movements) and amenorrhoea (lack of menstruation) in young women. This was thought to be due to it raising the patient's blood pressure. By the early 19th century, a second form of therapy had been developed, Faradism, that used induced electrical currents to treat all kinds of muscular paralysis. By the mid-19th century, a third application, electrolysis, had emerged. This was used to destroy naevuses and other skin deformities. Finally, in the 20th century, the thermal effects of high-frequency electrical currents found a use in surgery for stopping bleeding (diathermy), and from the 1950s electroconvulsive therapy became widely used as a treatment, initially for schizophrenia and later for severe depression.

Street and then right along City Road where you will see Wesley's chapel, designed by George Dance the Younger. Wesley lived in the house alongside, now a museum where his electrical machine can be seen in the first-floor drawing room of his house (www.wesleyschapel. org.uk).

Widespread enthusiasm for electrotherapy led to many establishments offering services. One such was the **London Electrical Dispensary**, established in a house on the other side of City Road in 1793 'with a view to afford a new benefit to the lower orders of mankind'. It survived for some 50 years. Continue along City Road, cross over and stop when you reach the roundabout.

In 1800 this was a simple crossroads. On the north side of the roundabout, on City Road where a fine red-stone Victorian building now stands, you would have seen one of the first hospitals to specialise in childbirth (p. 22) in London, the striking, neo-classical **City of London Hospital for Lying-In**. It had been founded in Aldersgate Street in 1750 and moved here in 1773 to custom-built premises designed by Robert Mylne. The eight wards, with eight beds in each, catered only for married women. As well as providing medical and midwifery care, the bonus of free baptisms on the last Sunday of every month was offered. Patients were received 'as near their time of reckoning as may be' and stayed for three weeks after delivery.

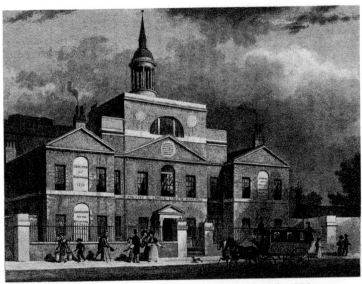

City of London Lying-In Hospital, designed by Robert Mylne in 1773, was damaged by the building of the Northern line in 1907 and by wartime bombing, which led to its closure and demolition in the 1950s

In 1907 the hospital was forced to rebuild because of damage caused by the building of the Northern line below City Road. Like so many other voluntary hospitals at the time, it included some pay-beds for more affluent patients as a way of boosting its income. During World War II, the building was bombed so inpatient care had to be moved to Brockett Hall, Hertfordshire. It never returned to City Road but was relocated to Crouch Hill, where it became part of the NHS. The original building here in City Road continued to provide outpatient care during the 1940s but was closed and demolished in the 1950s.

Standing here in 1800, you would have also seen, to the left of the Lying-In Hospital and extending nearly 200 m along Old Street, George Dance the Younger's palatial new home for **St Luke's Hospital**

for Lunatics. Built in 1786, it was a grand building, regarded as one of the architectural gems of London:

> *'there are few buildings in the metropolis, perhaps in Europe that, considering the poverty of the material (common English clamp bricks) possess such harmony of proportion with unity and appropriateness of style.'*

The vast frontage facing Old Street had a central entrance with the male wards to the left and female wards to the right. Behind the main building lay two airing yards where patients could exercise. The windows at the back of the building looked out, on the male side, upon a burial ground and Alleyn's Almshouses, while the women overlooked the Peerless Pool.

The interior was not quite so impressive – there were single 'cells' for the 300 patients, each with

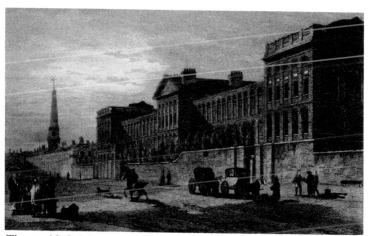

The second St Luke's Hospital for Lunatics, designed by George Dance the Younger in 1786, was thought to be one of the finest buildings in London. After the hospital closed in 1917, it became a print works, before being demolished in 1963

small windows set high in the wall and no heating, with loose straw on wooden bedsteads (although those deemed incurable only had straw). Large cold water baths (for shock therapy) were provided in the basements (and used until 1856). Otherwise treatment was focused on the gastrointestinal system: anti-spasmodics, emetics (to induce vomiting) and purgatives.

Despite the grandeur of the architecture, the building was uninviting, an impression Charles Dickens experienced when visiting on Boxing Day 1851:

> '*when on that cold, misty, cheerless afternoon I looked up at the high walls, and saw, grimly peering over them, its upper stories and dismal little iron-bound windows, I did not ring the porter's bell in the most cheerful frame of mind.*'

During the second half of the 19th century, various changes were made to make the interior less austere and cheerless. Despite such improvements, the building was by the start of the 20th century far from suitable for treating those who were mentally ill. After much deliberation the hospital closed, and the building was sold to the Bank of England in 1917 to be used as a print works. The building suffered some bomb damage from a German airship raid but continued to be used by the Bank until 1963, when it was deemed no longer suitable for any contemporary use and became another of the lost hospitals of St Luke's.

The walk ends here at Old Street underground station.

Walk 3: A cradle of reform

While health services are always changing, the middle decades of the 19th century were an extraordinarily active period of reform. And in Britain, one small area of St Pancras and Bloomsbury – bounded by Euston Road in the north, Gray's Inn Road in the east, Great Ormond Street in the south and Russell Square in the west – was to prove exceptionally influential. It may simply have been a coincidence that so many revolutionary changes emanated from this area between 1840 and 1880. But more likely the area attracted and accommodated reformers determined to challenge established ways and develop new health services, just as it has attracted reformers in fields as diverse as the penal system, adult education, literature and painting.

Between 1740 and 1840, as London spread north, the rural tranquillity of this area was replaced by terraced streets and squares. The only hospitals in the area were for those suffering infectious diseases – the London Smallpox Hospital and the London Fever Hospital – and for abandoned infants – the Foundling Hospital. Despite this, during the early decades of the 19th century, leading doctors and medical organisations had made the area just to the south, in Holborn, the centre of medical London.

The pace of change between 1840 and 1880 was remarkable. It was characterised by concern for those who had traditionally been ignored: children, who had largely been excluded from hospitals until the development of the Hospital for Sick Children and the Alexandra Hospital; the destitute poor (including those

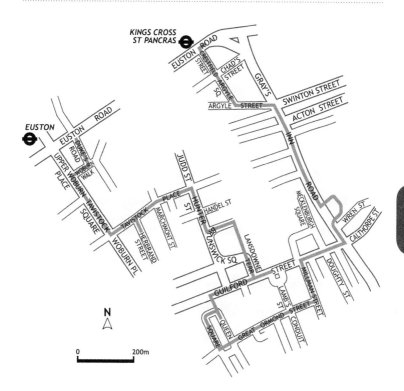

forced into prostitution), for whom the doors of the Royal Free Hospital were open; the aged and decrepit, cared for by the Hospital for Infirm and Incurable Women, the Hospital of St John & St Elizabeth, and Louisa Twining's Nursing Home for the Elderly & Epileptics; the paralysed and epileptic, for whom the Hospital for the Paralysed & Epileptic was created; pregnant women, largely excluded from general hospitals until the Royal Free Hospital established an obstetric service; and foreigners, such as Italians for whom the Ospedale Italiano was established.

It was not only patients who experienced the benefits of reform.

This area was also the birthplace of new opportunities for health care staff. It was here that women finally succeeded in storming the male medical establishment by creating the first medical school open to women and persuading a general hospital to provide clinical training for its students. And it was fitting that the first purpose-built hospital staffed by women and for women was established here. Conversely, the Hospital for the Paralysed & Epileptic was one of the first hospitals to employ male nurses in what had been an exclusively female preserve. The area also provided a home for a group of alternative practitioners that the medical establishment wanted outlawed in the 1850s, homeopaths. And the introduction of Lady Almoners (similar to modern-day hospital social workers) occurred here, in the Royal Free Hospital.

Alongside these major reforms, this walk also illustrates several other themes. First is the impact of the railways both in forcing hospitals to move as they were granted priority for land (London Smallpox Hospital, London Fever Hospital, Great Northern Hospital) and in increasing the accessibility of hospitals to those living outside London. Hospitals sited near stations, such as the Royal National Throat, Nose & Ear Hospital, gained an advantage over competitors.

Second, there was an often tricky relationship between doctors and managers. You will see the contrast between hospitals in which doctors have always participated and accepted some managerial responsibility (Royal National Throat, Nose & Ear Hospital, Royal Free Hospital, London Fever Hospital) and those in which the lay governors excluded doctors from management (Ospedale Italiano, National Hospital for the Paralysed & Epileptic). In the latter, tensions even led on occasion to mass medical resignations.

Third is the importance of international influences on health care: the introduction of smallpox inoculation from Turkey; the establishment of foundling hospitals modelled on those in Italy, Austria and Russia; the introduction of homeopathy from Germany; the creation of children's hospitals, copying those in France, Germany and Turkey; the training and employment of women doctors, which was already occurring in Italy, Germany and France; and the introduction of postgraduate education for doctors, already well established in Vienna and other European cities.

And finally, while most hospitals were founded by male doctors, some of the key developments in health services in this area of London were instigated by women doctors (Garrett Anderson's establishment of the New Hospital for Women), by nurses (Wood and colleagues who established the Alexandra Hospital) and by lay people (the Chandlers' establishment of the National Hospital for the Paralysed & Epileptic, Ortelli's founding of the Ospedale Italiano, Cardinal Wiseman's creation of the Hospital of St John & St Elizabeth).

With all these themes in mind, it is time to explore this area of London that was so influential in shaping health care, time to enter this cradle of reform. This walk starts at King's Cross underground station. Take the exit towards Euston Road (Southside). At the end of the tunnel under Euston Road, take the stairs to the left, emerging beside Crestfield Street. If you look back at the mainline station, you can see to its left the Great Northern Hotel, a curved Italianate building designed by Lewis Cubitt in 1854. It stands on the site of two infectious disease hospitals (p. 78) during the first half of the 19th century. The **London Smallpox Hospital** had been established near Tottenham Court Road in 1746 to treat and care for smallpox victims and provide

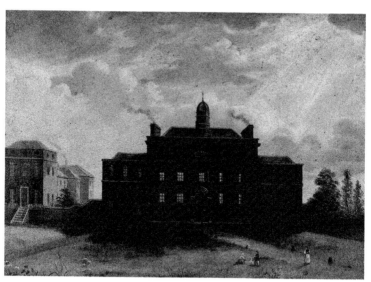

The governors of the London Smallpox Hospital commissioned this fine building in 1767 and, from 1815, accommodated the London Fever Hospital in the building to the left

inoculations (introduced to England from Turkey by a diplomat's wife in 1721). The hospital moved here in 1767, despite delays caused by objections and legal action taken by local residents who 'didn't want it in their backyard'. Initially, the hospital was restricted to inoculating people and keeping them under observation until the danger of them infecting others had passed. It was not until 1794 that more infectious 'casual' (naturally occurring) smallpox cases were allowed.

By 1800 the contagious nature of many infectious fevers was recognised. And when the upper classes realised that they too were endangered by such diseases of the poor, in particular from their own servants, action was finally taken. Influenced by the fever wards

and 'Houses of Recovery' already established in provincial towns, the 'Fever Hospital Movement' founded the **London Fever Hospital** in 1801, about 100 m south of here on Gray's Inn Road. Again, the hospital was not welcomed by local residents, who feared its presence. Increasing demand for admission meant that its 15 beds soon proved inadequate, so in 1815 it moved into a building alongside the Smallpox Hospital, here at King's Cross.

It was not public concern but the coming of the railways that led to both hospitals having to move from here. Relatively large sites were needed in London to construct stations, sidings and all the associated buildings needed to handle passengers and freight. In 1848 the Great Northern Railway

Infectious disease hospitals

The first hospitals for infectious disease were for leprosy (p. 17), of which there were ten around the outskirts of London. Established as religious institutions from about 1100, the last one closed in the 16th century with the disappearance of leprosy. Some were subsequently used in the 17th century as pest houses to isolate and confine the victims of plague.

From about 1700 the greatest fear was smallpox, which although endemic (ever present) also caused frequent epidemics. Inoculation, in which infected material from a smallpox victim was injected to try to cause only a mild illness, was introduced in 1721 but proved to be too risky. Even when replaced with a milder inoculation in the 1740s, full-blown smallpox could still result. The London Smallpox Hospital, established in 1746, moved in 1753 to Coldbath Fields. This accommodation proved inadequate and was replaced with a purpose-built hospital at King's Cross in 1767. The replacement of inoculation with much safer vaccination (using lymph from cows with cowpox) from 1799 led to the creation of the National Vaccine Establishment in 1809 in Fitzrovia to ensure and maintain lymph supplies.

Meanwhile, concern about other infectious diseases (which both voluntary general hospitals and workhouse infirmaries did not admit) led to the establishment of the Institution for the Cure and Prevention of Contagious Fevers in 1801 in Gray's Inn Road. After unsuccessful attempts to move to Coldbath Fields, it moved in 1815 into a building beside the Smallpox Hospital at King's Cross as the London Fever Hospital. The coming of the railways meant that both had to move again in 1848, the Smallpox Hospital migrating to Highgate and the Fever Hospital to Islington.

The need for greater coordination and planning of hospital services for infectious diseases was one of the reasons for the establishment of the Metropolitan Asylums Board (p. 179) in 1867. Over the following ten years, five fever hospitals were built on the outskirts of London, and five more were added in the 1890s following the decision to allow non-paupers as well as paupers to be admitted. This integrated system was supplemented in the 1880s by the commissioning of hospital ships on the Thames, replaced around 1900 by a huge complex (the River Hospitals) constructed near Dartford, Kent. London's ability to deal with major infectious disease outbreaks had finally been achieved just as the threat from smallpox was disappearing (partly thanks to almost 50 years of compulsory vaccination of infants).

The new challenges were TB (p. 218) and venereal diseases (p. 123). During the early decades of the 20th century, the Metropolitan Asylums Board oversaw the development of TB sanatoria (in addition to those created by voluntary hospitals) outside London.

Meanwhile, within London the Board established two hospitals for venereal diseases to supplement the voluntary specialist hospitals that existed.

By the 1940s, with the advent of antibiotics and vaccines, the threat of infectious diseases was receding, and the need for specialist hospitals, such as the London Fever Hospital, lessened as general hospitals created isolation facilities to enable them to admit such patients.

identified the site it required to build King's Cross Station, an area largely taken up by the Great Dust Heap, a mountain of ashes from domestic and industrial fires that was dumped here to be used with local clay for brick-making. However, the required land also included the Smallpox Hospital and the Fever Hospital. They and the Great Dust Heap were duly removed, the latter (it is alleged) being used to help rebuild the city of Moscow. A new Smallpox and Vaccination Hospital was constructed in Highgate (now part of the Whittington Hospital), while the London Fever Hospital moved to Islington.

By the middle of the 19th century, this area was already densely populated, deprived and rather unsalubrious, being known as 'Shadyville'. The only health care for the sick poor (apart from the local workhouse infirmary) was the Royal Free Hospital (about 700 m to the south) which had opened in 1842. Recognising the inadequate provision for local people, a young physician working at University College Hospital, Sherard Statham, established the **Great Northern Hospital** in 1856. It was located in a house to the right of the station in York Way, similar to those that you can see today. Like so many small voluntary hospitals, it was founded by a doctor who felt he was a victim of medical nepotism and corruption in the voluntary general hospital (p. 148) in which he worked. What was unusual in this case was that he created a small general hospital; it was more usual for such people to create specialist hospitals, some examples of which you will see on this walk.

The Great Northern Hospital initially had 16 beds. Unlike most voluntary hospitals, patients did not need a letter of recommendation from a subscriber. Not surprisingly, there was great demand for its services so that it had to expand into two adjacent houses and some workshops. It survived the construction of the mainline station, but the extension of the Metropolitan line in 1861 meant the hospital had to move. After three years in temporary accommodation, the hospital found a new home on Caledonian Road before moving again in 1888, this time to Holloway (later becoming the Royal Northern Hospital and finally, in 1982, part of the Whittington Hospital).

Walk away from Euston Road along Crestfield Street and through

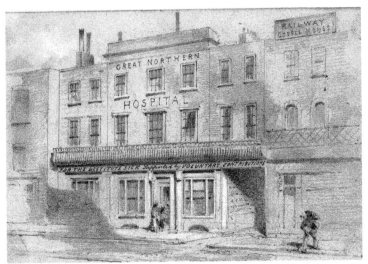

The Great Northern Hospital was established in houses alongside King's Cross station in 1856, but construction of the Metropolitan line soon forced it to move

Argyle Square, where you can see some of the grander houses from the 19th century. At the end turn left into Argyle Street. After 100 m you will reach Gray's Inn Road. On the opposite side, to your left, is the **Royal National Throat, Nose & Ear Hospital**, one of many voluntary specialist hospitals (p. 119) established during the second half of the 19th century.

It was founded in 1874 by Lennox Browne, a surgeon from one of the three ENT hospitals (p. 82) that existed in London at the time, located in Golden Square, Soho. For its first three years, this new establishment was simply a dispensary in a house in Argyle Street (which you have just walked along). The hospital then acquired two houses on Gray's Inn Road (similar to those alongside you) and replaced them with a new 15-bed

hospital, the façade of which you can see, despite the rather unsympathetic entrance that was added in the 1970s. The original design, influenced by Nightingale and other sanitarians, included noiseless window sashes and glazed tiles on internal walls.

Its success over the following century can be attributed to four factors. First, its location near the railway stations attracted patients from afar: in the first four days patients arrived from Cambridge, Carlisle, Hull and Liverpool. Second, unlike some voluntary hospitals, doctors were involved and represented on the management committee. This helped to avoid the sort of event that occurred at the ENT hospital in Golden Square, where four senior doctors resigned in 1887 when governors insisted they sign an attendance book. Third, the hospital

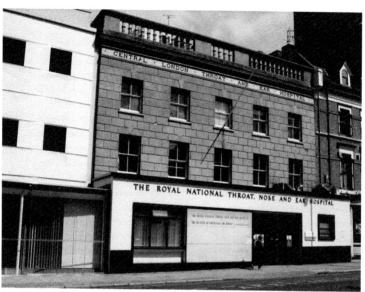

The Central London Throat & Ear Hospital, built in 1877, which was to become the largest ENT hospital in the world, unfortunately defaced its original building with the addition of an unsympathetic modern entrance

was unique in developing specialist training for doctors and nurses. And fourth, with foresight the governors bought up adjacent properties as they became available (including a church, school, cottages and a print works), thus ensuring they would have the capacity to host any future merger of ENT hospitals (although this was not to occur until the 1940s). Its pre-eminent position was confirmed when the University of London established its postgraduate institute (p. 101) for laryngology and otology here in 1949. Further additions, including the recent building to the left of the original hospital, have resulted in it becoming the largest ENT hospital in the world.

Turn right and walk along Gray's Inn Road. On the other side of the road, you will see a modern office building, home of the National Union of Journalists, which is on the site of the original home of the **London Fever Hospital**. Continue for another 400 m until you reach an old granite water trough for horses, opposite the old **Royal Free Hospital**.

In 1828 William Marsden, a surgeon, organised a meeting in Gray's Inn Coffee House where he laid out his plans to establish a hospital that would offer free care to anybody. Existing voluntary general hospitals required patients to have a letter of recommendation from a subscriber to gain admission. Marsden was motivated by finding a young girl dying of disease and hunger on the steps of a Holborn church. Three

ENT hospitals

In 1816, John Harrison Curtis, a retired naval surgeon with no recognised medical qualifications, established the first successful voluntary specialist hospital (p. 119) for ear disease, the Dispensary for Diseases of the Ear. This met with opposition from licensed doctors who thought that such self-designated aurists were putting off qualified doctors from specialising in the area. The situation was aggravated in 1822 when the King approved its designation as the Royal Dispensary for Diseases of the Ear.

The first institution set up by a surgeon was the Metropolitan Institution for Diseases of the Eye & Ear established in 1838 by James Yearsley in Piccadilly. The combination of eyes and ears was not new: John Cunningham Saunders had created the London Dispensary for Curing Diseases of the Eye and Ear in 1805, but within three years it had become an eye hospital. In contrast, in 1848 Yearsley chose to focus on ears.

It was not until 1860 that another ENT hospital appeared, but over the following 27 years the pattern of specialist services for London was set. In 1860 the Metropolitan Free Dispensary for Diseases of the Throat & Loss of Voice was established by Morrell Mackenzie near Regent Street, before moving to Golden Square in 1865. In 1877 it was renamed the Hospital for Diseases of the Throat & Chest, around the same time two other hospitals were founded: the Municipal Infirmary for Diseases of the Throat in City Road and the Central London Throat & Ear Hospital. The latter started as a dispensary, but within a year it moved to custom-built premises in Gray's Inn Road and was renamed the Central London Throat, Nose & Ear Hospital. Meanwhile, in 1875, the Metropolitan Institution had moved from Piccadilly to Fitzrovia. The final specialist hospital to be established was the London Throat Hospital in Great Portland Street in 1887.

By the early 20th century, voluntary general hospitals (p. 148) recognised the need to include specialist services for ear, nose and throat conditions. Up until then such cases had been treated by general surgeons. There was also pressure from bodies such as the Ministry of Health and the King's Fund for the various ENT hospitals to amalgamate, but the hospitals were wary of such moves as they each feared for their own survival. Recognising that mergers would eventually occur, the Central London in Gray's Inn Road embarked on a policy of acquiring land so it would be able to expand to include the other hospitals. After 1913 the pattern of services altered radically: one hospital closed (the Municipal Infirmary in 1927); two merged with general hospitals (the Royal Ear with University College Hospital in 1920 and the Metropolitan Institution with Charing Cross Hospital in 1985); and three coalesced: the London Throat and the Hospital for Diseases of the Throat & Chest merged in 1913, and these then merged with the Central London in 1942 to become the Royal National Throat, Nose & Ear Hospital. It remained on two sites until 1985, when services at Golden Square transferred to Gray's Inn Road.

hospitals had refused her admission so he cared for in lodgings near his home. Two days later she died 'unrecognised by any human being'. He determined to establish a hospital 'to which the only passport should be poverty and disease'.

Seven weeks after the coffee house meeting, the London General Institution for the Gratuitous Cure of Malignant Diseases opened in Hatton Garden. Unlike many hospitals, it remained open during the cholera epidemic. In 1833 it was renamed the London Free Hospital, and four years later, having received Queen Victoria's endorsement, it acquired its permanent title of Royal Free Hospital. It was to be the most radical and innovatory of the 12 London teaching hospitals, reflecting the motivation and aim of its founder.

In 1842 the governors acquired the lease on the abandoned barracks of the Light Horse Volunteers here in Gray's Inn Road. Built around a quadrangle, it boasted a grand entrance arch surmounted by a British lion. Initially, the existing buildings designed for accommodating horses rather than people were used, but the buildings were gradually replaced or enhanced. In 1856 the north wing was rebuilt (Sussex Wing, the end of which can be seen on the left), and then in 1876 the south wing (Victoria Wing, to the right of the main entrance), and finally the west wing with its frontage onto Gray's Inn Road was rebuilt in 1893 (Alexandra Building).

The hospital's commitment to Marsden's radicalism can be seen in several ways. First, by its provision of care to those in need irrespective of their circumstances, it treated people that other hospitals turned away. A subscriber's letter was not needed, and even patients with venereal disease were accepted; as a consequence, prostitutes were admitted:

'These poor girls, enticed from their country homes, seduced,

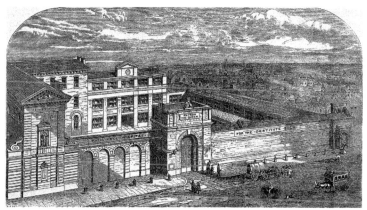

The Royal Free Hospital in 1856, when it was still largely using abandoned military barracks except for the newly built Sussex Wing, on the left

diseased, abandoned, distant from all early and better influences, have no shelter or refuge left to them save within the walls of institutions similar to the Royal Free.'

Second, in 1877 it agreed to provide access for clinical teaching to students from the nearby London School of Medicine for Women (which you will see later on this walk). Apart from a brief period during World War I and a small annual quota at University College, it was the only hospital in London to accept female medical students before 1947.

Third, in 1895 it was the first hospital to appoint a Lady Almoner, Miss Mary Stewart, whose job was 'to ensure that patients in poor

circumstances were helped to benefit from treatments recommended by medical staff and to prevent the abuse of the hospital by persons able to pay for medical treatment'. Although she focused more on the former than the latter, the public perceived her as a threat, fearful that she would attempt to collect money from them. And the doctors resented her 'interference' in patient selection. Despite this, she became known as 'Lady Harmony', and over the following eight years six other hospitals appointed a Lady Almoner, all of whom were 'trained' by Mary Stewart. An exception was St Mary's Hospital in Paddington, which, more concerned about stopping abuse of its charity than assisting the poor, appointed an

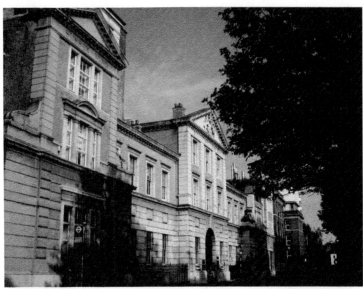

The three main wings of the former Royal Free Hospital. From left to right: the end of the Sussex Wing (1856); the Alexandra Wing, containing the main entrance (1893); and the end of Victoria Wing (1876)

Lady Almoners

While demand for inpatient care in voluntary general hospitals (p. 148) was limited by bed availability, there was no limit on outpatient attendances. In theory, attendance at most hospitals required a letter of recommendation from a subscriber, but in practice free care was sometimes provided for those without a letter. By 1870 many subscribers (and the British Medical Association) believed that charity was being abused, which harmed the hospitals and was deemed to have 'a demoralising effect on the perpetrators'. Charles Loch of the Charities Organisation Society, established in 1869 to coordinate hospital charities, felt that charities were 'helping to thrust a man into the great decadent class to which eventually the word "pauper" is applied'.

In 1871 the voluntary hospitals started encouraging those who could afford it to contribute to insurance schemes run by Friendly Societies, churches and other organisations, or to join a provident dispensary (p. 229). The Royal Free Hospital reckoned that 40% of people could afford to join such a scheme. In addition, hospitals needed a means of discriminating between those who lacked means and those who lacked self-respect, a task that 'ought not to be entrusted to the hall porter'.

In 1895 the Royal Free agreed to a three-month experiment of having a trained social worker 'to prevent abuse by those who could afford to pay, to refer those in need of relief to the Poor Law, and to recommend all who could afford to do so to join a provident dispensary'. Thus, the first Lady Almoner, Mary Stewart, came into being. The title was based on that used by governors at St Bartholomew's and St Thomas' in their role of selecting patients worthy of receiving alms.

Reactions were mixed. The public perceived the role as being associated with collecting money, and the doctors resented Stewart's interference in patient selection, complaining that she excluded many who were valuable for teaching (and as such, a source of personal income to doctors). In contrast, encouragement to pursue this initiative came from one important source of funding voluntary hospitals (p. 159), the Hospital Saturday Fund.

Over the following eight years, six other London hospitals appointed a Lady Almoner, although not all subscribed to the Stewart approach, which sought to assess patients' needs rather than their means. In contrast, St Mary's Hospital appointed a retired policeman because it was believed his experience of spotting criminals was ideal for 'protecting the hospital from exploitation'.

In 1920 the almoners formed their own Association, but two years later another organisation, the Institute of Hospital Almoners, was created. Whether intended or not, the latter served to limit (female) almoners' aspirations as they were outnumbered two to one by (male) representatives of charities, hospital governors and doctors. The professionalisation of almoners was delayed until 1946, when the two bodies merged. With universal access to free treatment in the NHS, almoners could focus entirely on patients' needs rather than their means, a role supported even by the Royal College of Physicians. Thus, modern medical social work was born.

ex-policeman on the grounds that he was skilled in spotting miscreants.

And fourth, in 1918 it was the first voluntary general hospital in modern times to provide lying-in care for childbirth (p. 22). And all these extraordinary innovations were made despite it being the poorest of the 12 teaching hospitals in London.

After World War II (during which the Victoria Wing suffered bomb damage), the drive to move some teaching hospitals out of central London gathered pace. After much discussion, it was decided to rebuild the Royal Free in Hampstead, a move that eventually took place in 1974. The old building was taken over in 1988 by the **Eastman Dental Hospital**, which had started as the dental department of the Royal Free Hospital. (If the large entrance doors are open, you

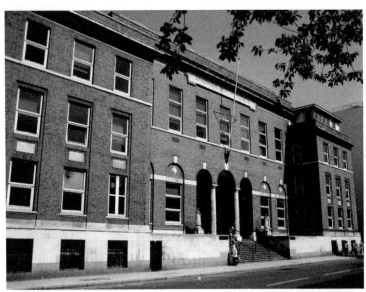

The Eastman Dental Clinic, built in 1929 as the dental department of the Royal Free Hospital, gained independence in 1948

can wander into the quadrangle and see the 19th century buildings.)

Continue along Gray's Inn Road and stop after 100 m opposite the entrance to the original Eastman Dental Hospital. It was built on the site of a munitions factory in 1929, funded by an American, George Eastman of Eastman Kodak, to provide dental care for poor children. Having lost his own teeth early in life and with a lifelong concern for the health of children (perhaps fuelled by being a childless bachelor himself), his hope was that 'eventually the poor will be able to chaw their food as well as the rich'. This was the first of five dental clinics he established in European capitals between 1929 and 1935. Sensitive to children's fear of dentistry, the waiting room housed a large, central bird-cage to entertain the young patients.

In 1948 the dental department separated from the Royal Free Hospital to become an independent hospital. Its main purpose changed from routine treatment to receiving referrals for specialist treatment, a change that was supported by the University of London, which established its postgraduate institute for dental surgery here. The hospital's expansion in the 1990s into the old Royal Free Hospital building was aided by the closure of University College Dental Hospital, near Tottenham Court Road.

Cross Gray's Inn Road and immediately beyond the Eastman Dental Hospital enter St Andrew's Gardens, the site of a disused graveyard. On entering, stop after

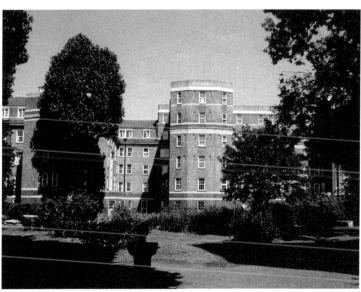

The Alfred Langton Nurses' Home, built in 1925 by the Royal Free Hospital, was one of many huge nurses' homes built at that time

50 m at the public drinking fountain, one of many set up in the 19th century to provide clean water for the poor.

Beyond the gardens, you will see the back of a large brick building, one of many large nurses' homes (p. 151) built by voluntary hospitals in the first half of the 20th century. The Alfred Langton Nurses' Home, built by the Royal Free Hospital, opened in 1925 and provided 'everything for the convenience and comfort of nurses'. Since the hospital's move to Hampstead, the home has become a hall of residence for university students.

Turn right and follow the path through the gardens and exit onto Gray's Inn Road. Turn left and walk 50 m to the junction with Calthorpe Street. The corner house on the other side of Calthorpe Street was, for 77 years, the home of a leading eye hospital (p. 59), the **Central London Ophthalmic Hospital**.

Eye disease was a common reason for establishing specialist hospitals and dispensaries in the 19th century. This, the fourth in London, was established in 1843. As with other specialist institutions, the founder was a doctor, Alfred Smee. By the early 1900s, the

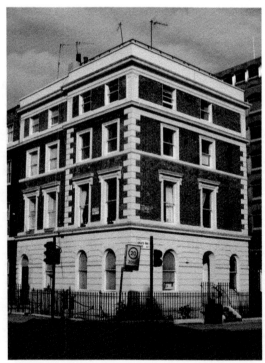

The home of the Central London Ophthalmic Hospital from its establishment in 1843 until 1925, one of the leading eye hospitals in London

accommodation was proving to be inadequate, so the governors suggested a merger with the other eye hospitals in central London. The Royal London Ophthalmic Hospital, which had recently moved to City Road, 'entertained no idea of amalgamation'. Faced with no prospect of an imminent merger, the Central London moved in 1925 to custom-built premises in Judd Street (which you will visit later on this walk).

Cross Gray's Inn Road and then cross Guilford Street and proceed along it. You are now entering an area in which child health and welfare has been a major concern over the past 250 years. The first indications are evident from the plaques on houses on the left as you walk along: No. 6 was the home of **St Nicholas Nursery** from 1954 to 1964 (run in association with the Hospital for Sick Children), and (after crossing Doughty Street) at No. 10 the **Sick Children's Trust** provides free accommodation for the families of children in the nearby hospital. As you turn left into Millman Street, note the 1950s' building on the opposite side of the road that housed the headquarters of the British Postgraduate Medical

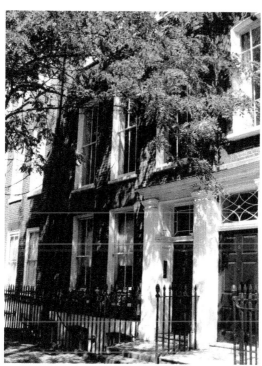

The Hospital for Infirm & Incurable Women was established in this 18th century townhouse (with the blue door) in 1861. It moved to Finchley in 1889

Federation from 1955 until the 1990s, this being responsible for the 14 postgraduate institutes spread across London.

After about 150 m, take the road on the right, Great Ormond Street. Unlike further on, this first part of Great Ormond Street is largely unchanged from the 19th century. No. 10 (a few doors along on the right) was the **Hospital for Infirm & Incurable Women**, a title that patients today might find rather discouraging. In modern terms, this was a nursing home with a Lady Resident, Mrs Bettison, and honorary medical staff available when required. Established in 1861, it provided care for 32 women who would not have been welcome in the general hospitals as they were unlikely to recover. In 1889 the hospital moved to the more rural environs of Woodside, near Finchley.

Cross Great Ormond Street and continue along it, stopping after crossing Lamb's Conduit Street. In the mid-19th century, this part of Great Ormond Street was lined by fine Georgian terraced houses, some of which survive on the left (south) side. Between 1850 and 1920, the Hospital for Sick Children acquired all the properties (Nos 41–49) on the north side, gradually demolishing them to make way for new hospital buildings.

One of those lost was No. 44, which was the **Hospital for Sick Children's Private Nurses' House**. A key component of the transformation of nursing during the second half of the 19th century was the establishment of nursing schools by voluntary hospitals. Hospitals needed well-trained nurses not only for their inpatients, but also for their 'nursing institutions', which generated income by hiring out nurses to upper- and middle-class patients. When not hired out, the nurses lived in the nursing institution. Demand for this service extended to well outside London, as illustrated by Dr Moon of Broadstairs, who reported:

> *'When I have an ill child in my practice and the whole household is in hysterics – I telephone to Miss Thomas for help. She sends me down one of her pink nurses [from the Hospital for Sick Children] and within the hour peace is restored and the patient is asleep.'*

Before its acquisition by the Hospital for Sick Children, No. 47 was the **Hospital of St John & St Elizabeth**. It was founded in 1856 by Cardinal Wiseman and Sisters of Mercy nurses returning from the Crimean War. Like its neighbour at No. 10, it catered for women suffering from incurable or long-standing disease. The accommodation proved increasingly cramped, and they transferred to a new building in St John's Wood in 1901. But not only the hospital moved. The church of St John & St Elizabeth, next door at No. 46, was also moved, brick by brick, and re-erected at their new home, where 'John & Lizzie's' has become the third largest private acute hospital in the UK.

Walk on along Great Ormond Street and stop opposite Powis

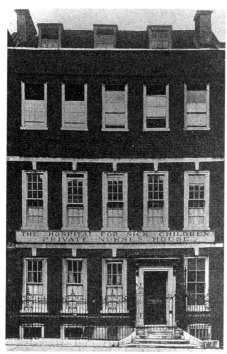

The Hospital for Sick Children Private Nurses' House provided accommodation for nurses when they were not hired out to private patients

Place. Until the middle of the 19th century, there was little hospital care available for children. Despite half of all deaths occurring in childhood and several books on childhood diseases having been published in the 18th century, children made up only 6% of inpatients in the voluntary general hospitals in London. Lack of hospital provision was justified on the grounds that the care of children was best left to mothers. Indeed, many believed it would be wrong to separate children from mothers by admitting them to hospital. In addition, the poor survival of children in the Foundling Hospital (only 4,400 of the initial 15,000

survived) suggested that there were dangers in institutionalising them. The absence of a children's hospital in London was in sharp contrast to its European neighbours. The Hôpital des Enfants Malades had been established in Paris in 1802, and similar institutions existed in Germany, Italy, Russia, Austria, Denmark and Turkey.

In 1849 Charles West resigned as a physician at one of the few dispensaries (p. 229) devoted to children, the Universal Dispensary for Children in Waterloo, and galvanised a group of aristocrats including Lord Byron's wife and daughter, Baroness Burdett-Coutts (the richest woman in England) and Lord Shaftesbury to raise funds for a children's hospital. No. 49 Great Ormond Street, a fine Queen Anne-style end-of-terrace house on the corner of Powis Place, was purchased, and the **Hospital for Sick Children** opened in 1852. The trepidation of mothers in bringing their sick children was not to be easily overcome. It was to be the social reformer Charles Dickens who, writing an article entitled 'Drooping buds' in his popular magazine *Household Words*, provided the reassurance mothers sought.

Despite acquiring a convalescent home (p. 92) in Highgate to relieve the pressure on beds, the need to expand persisted and led to the purchase of No. 48 next door. Both houses had large gardens, which, in 1875, provided the land for the construction of Edward Barry's 'Hospital in the Gardens', a Victorian red-brick gothic building that included a Byzantine-style chapel. All that remains of the building, which faced onto Powis Place, is the south wing (in front of you). The chapel survives (having been moved 18 m on hydraulic skates

Convalescent homes

While some voluntary hospitals in the late 18th century had convalescent wards, as did some workhouse infirmaries (p. 54) in the early 19th century, the first convalescent home was not established until 1841. Nightingale, a strong advocate of convalescent homes, felt they should be domestic in style, ideally a group of cottages. It took time for the idea to be accepted, and while some were small and homely, many built in the late 19th century were huge edifices. The attraction to hospitals was the prospect of freeing beds, thus increasing income, while patients benefited from the fresh air and sea-water available on the south and east coasts, popular locations for homes.

Initially, they tended to be similar in design to hospitals, reflecting their curative role (particularly for TB) as much as their convalescent role. They were usually managed by nurses who could call on local private doctors if medical advice was needed. It was not only voluntary hospitals that created homes, but also Poor Law Unions, the Metropolitan Asylums Board (p. 179) and membership organisations such as Friendly Societies, Working Men's Clubs and trades unions. Most of those established by hospitals closed before or soon after the establishment of the NHS, although the rest survived longer. Their demise resulted from improvements in the home conditions of patients, in the provision of domiciliary health and social care, and in the development of local authority residential facilities, and from a perception that the need for them had passed.

over the course of two days in the 1990s) and can be visited if you go in through the modern main entrance and follow the signs.

Over the following 100 years, the hospital expanded. First, in 1908 the neighbouring two houses in Great Ormond Street, where the present-day entrance is, were bought and demolished to make way for a new outpatient department, which in turn was demolished. Next, in 1920 a suggestion to relocate to a 'country hospital city' 30 miles from London was made but failed to materialise. Instead, in Powis Place, the north wing of Barry's building made way in 1938 for a huge new building along the northern side of the site, the Southwood Building, which had extensive balconies for nursing children in the open air. You can see part of this building at the far end of Powis Place, although in 2012 its future is threatened by further redevelopment. (In the 1950s, Powis Place was the scene of an extraordinary daily event. To maximise its use as a doctors' car park, a turntable was installed at the far end so drivers did not have to reverse out. One doctor, Robert Beaver, perfected the art of driving in at high speed such that when he stopped suddenly on the turntable, it would rotate automatically.)

In the 1990s another portion of the Barry building was demolished

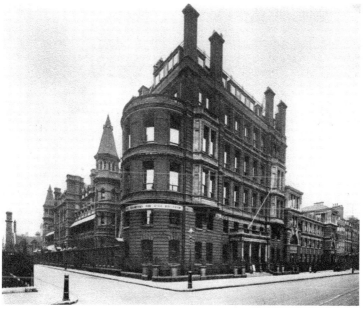

The 'Hospital in the Gardens' extending along Powis Place was designed by Edward Barry in 1875 for the Hospital for Sick Children. The southern wing (on Great Ormond Street in the foreground), designed by his brother Charles, was not completed until 1893 and is all that survives

to make way for a large new building extending through the centre of the site. To learn more about the Hospital for Sick Children, you can visit its museum at No. 55 (by appointment; 020 7405 9200 ext 5920).

To the left of Powis Place, you will see the **Royal London Homeopathic Hospital**. This is a testament to the success of homeopaths in their battles with established medicine in the mid-19th century. At that time, the medical profession (p. 200) was seeking to establish a monopoly in the face of a plethora of alternative medical approaches, including homeopathy. The latter was deemed an 'absurd system' by the President of the Royal College of Physicians, a body that wanted homeopaths outlawed by the 1858 Medical Act.

The foreign origins of homeopathy, centred on Germany, may have contributed to the hostility. Part of the reason medical opposition failed was the support that homeopathy enjoyed from aristocrats and royalty, support that continues to this day.

Like other voluntary specialist hospitals, it was founded by an enthusiastic physician, Frederick Quinn, a wit and raconteur much admired in the highest social circles. With the hospital established in Golden Square, Soho in 1850, he claimed that only 16% of its cholera patients died during an epidemic compared with 52% at other voluntary hospitals. The hospital moved to three houses in Great Ormond Street in 1859, these being replaced in 1895 by the building you see today.

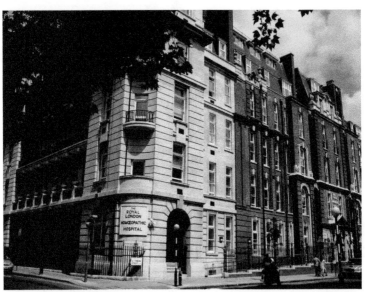

The Royal London Homeopathic Hospital, built in 1895 in Great Ormond Street (on the right), with the large 1911 white stone extension with balconies (on the left) overlooking Queen Square

Interest in homeopathy has varied over the years, enjoying a heyday in the 1930s and 40s (culminating in 1948 when the Queen became patron, it gained its 'Royal' designation and it was incorporated into the NHS) and again since the 1980s. Recognising the potential benefits of other alternative and complementary systems, the hospital has now diversified to also include acupuncture and other approaches. Interest in and demand for such therapies is reflected in its redesignation in 2010 as the Royal London Hospital for Integrated Care, focused entirely on outpatient care.

Continue to the end of Great Ormond Street, passing on your left Weston House, a six-storey red-brick and stone building built in 1912 as a nurses' home for the Homeopathic Hospital, but acquired and renovated by the Hospital for Sick Children in 2005 to be a 'patient hotel', providing accommodation for patients and their families.

Cross over to the 18th century public water pump in Queen Square. There is no other location in London so steeped in the history of health care. Standing here in 1885 you would have seen seven hospitals, a sight unequalled anywhere else in the world. Robert Louis Stevenson observed that Queen Square seemed to have been set aside for 'the humanities of life and alleviation of all hard destinies'.

If you look back towards Great Ormond Street, you can see to the left the large white stone extension to the Royal London Homeopathic

Hospital, built in 1911. To your right, on the short side of the square, is the former **Ospedale Italiano**, one of several hospitals established in London to provide health care for foreigners (p. 19). Unlike most specialist hospitals, it was not established by a doctor but by a lay person, Commendatore Giovanni Ortelli, a resident Italian businessman. In 1884 he donated two houses (similar to those adjoining it), which were demolished in 1898 to make way for the building you see today. It was extended in 1910 when two houses behind the hospital were acquired.

Unlike many voluntary specialist hospitals, management was in the hands of lay governors, an approach that at times led to friction with the medical staff. For example, in 1935 all the doctors resigned when they felt the governors were appointing clinical staff without suitable qualifications.

The façade carried the inscription, 'Charity knows no restriction of country', and this was apparent in the clientele, half of whom were British rather than Italian. Funds were raised from subscribers not only in Britain, but also in Italy. Among the former, during the 1930s, were British Fascists whose admiration for Benito Mussolini extended to their endowing a bed dedicated to Il Duce. Despite a common purpose, tension between the Italian and British governors existed. This culminated in the British resigning in 1937 in protest at the demand by some Italian members to have more

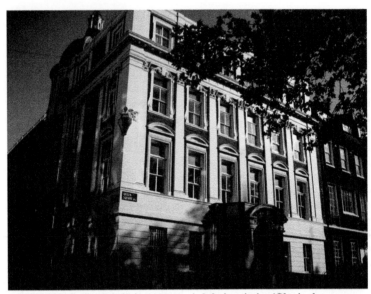

The Ospedale Italiano, built in 1898, carried the inscription 'Charity knows no restriction of country'. On closing in 1990, the building was acquired by Great Ormond Street Hospital

control. The onset of World War II led to closure of the hospital, but it reopened in 1948 and continued as an independent institution until 1990. The building was acquired by the Hospital for Sick Children for offices and facilities for staff.

Walk along the left side of the garden in the square. On your left you pass a pub, the Queens' Larder, with a notice explaining one of the square's earliest connections with health care. A few doors further on (Nos 8–11) is Sir Charles Symonds House, built in 1912 as the **Conjoint Examination Hall** for the two medical royal colleges (p. 194) that existed at that time. Their coats of arms can be seen on the façade. It served this function until the late 1980s, when the 'conjoint exam', an alternative to a university medical degree as an entry to medicine, ceased. The building was sold to the National Hospital for Neurology & Neurosurgery (see below).

The next few properties include three important contributions to the history of nursing. First, at No. 12 you will see **St John's House**, built in 1906 as the headquarters for the famous nursing sisterhood (p. 163) that transformed the running of King's College Hospital in 1856 and, a decade later, Charing Cross Hospital.

Walk on to the end of the square, noting the three Georgian houses (Nos 13–15) that give an idea of how the square looked before it was taken over by doctors and hospitals. The last building, Alexandra House, was

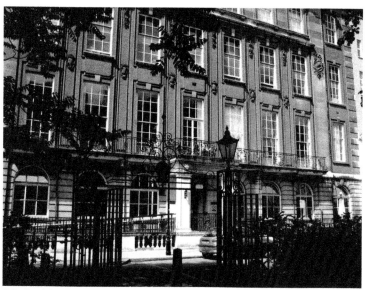

The Conjoint Examination Hall built in 1912 for the Royal Colleges of Physicians and of Surgeons, whose coats of arms can be seen on the façade, in which exams to gain a medical qualification were held until the late 1980s

until 1920 the **Alexandra Hospital for Children with Hip Disease**. Its establishment in 1867 is noteworthy as it was the first hospital in London to be founded by nurses, including Catherine Wood, the most senior nurse at the Hospital for Sick Children. The hospital focused on tuberculosis (p. 218) of the hip, a common disease in children at the time. As with most specialist hospitals, it outgrew its initial townhouse accommodation, which was replaced in 1899 to make way for the building you see today. It also made use of convalescent homes in Bournemouth, Gloucestershire and Surrey. The hospital itself moved out of central London in 1920 and survived until 1958. The building here was initially converted to offices before being

acquired by the National Hospital for Neurology & Neurosurgery.

In the 19th century, there were two more houses beyond the Alexandra Hospital, in the first of which (No. 20, demolished in 1960) Louisa Twining, one of the most effective social reformers of the 19th century, lived from 1866 to 1882 and ran a **Nursing Home for Elderly and for Epileptics**. Over the preceding two decades, she had irritated the authorities by publicising the appalling state of workhouse infirmaries (p. 54) and, in particular, the lack of trained nurses. In 1879 the Association for Promoting Trained Nurses in Workhouse Infirmaries was created, and by 1898 it had trained and placed 800 nurses.

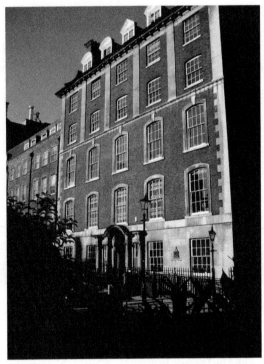

The Alexandra Hospital for Children with Hip Disease, founded by nurses in 1867, occupied townhouses on this site until replaced by this building in 1899. It moved out of London in 1920, surviving until 1958

Walk along the short side of the square. The building on this side of the square (No. 23) was built for the Royal Institute of Public Health, an independent body established in 1892 to promote public health. On either side of the entrance is a lamp on top of a caduceus (a staff and two entwined snakes), the symbol of Hermes, conductor of the dead and protector of merchants and thieves! This is not the only medical organisation to mistake the caduceus for the staff of Aesclepius, the god of healing, which has only one entwined snake. The original

perpetrator of this error seems to have been the medical department of the US Army in 1902. The building is now part of the Institute of Neurology.

When you reach the corner, turn right and stop by the garden railings in front of the main entrance to the **National Hospital of Neurology & Neurosurgery**, the first hospital to be established in the square. Before the middle of the 19th century, there were no facilities for the care and treatment of those with neurological conditions causing paralysis and epilepsy. The lack of medical interest in such conditions reflected fear and ignorance, the absence of any effective treatments and the impoverished state of many sufferers, making this an unprofitable area in which to specialise. Until the Poor Law was amended in 1867, those with epilepsy and those who were paralysed were consigned to the 'insane' wards of workhouses. It is therefore not surprising that, unlike almost all other specialist hospitals and dispensaries, the first institution devoted to the paralysed and epileptic was founded not by doctors but by lay people – Johanna, Louisa and Edward Chandler – who had cared for their paralysed grandmother.

The National Hospital for the Paralysed & Epileptic opened in two houses on this site in 1860 with space for 36 inpatients and providing therapies based on water and on electricity (p. 69). It was not universally welcomed by its neighbours, who objected to patients walking or sitting in the gardens. In response, patients took chairs and sat at the end of the square outside the railings of Queen Square House (now the site of Queen Court mansion block to your left), much to the displeasure of the resident, the Lord Chief Justice.

The key role of lay people in its foundation continued in its management, with the attendant tensions between lay governors and medical staff. The former were adamant that if doctors were included in management, 'the hospital would be in danger of having the philanthropic aspect of its

work subordinated to that which is merely scientific and investigatory', concerns that resonate with some politicians and patient organisations today. There is some suggestion that the governors' fears were well placed. In 1869 a visiting German doctor, Dr Pelman, recognised that the hospital was 'a pure jewel-case ... containing beautiful baths of every kind, including, naturally, a Turkish bath; a spacious room very richly equipped with electrical fittings, and an impressive gymnasium' but observed that it was not apparent that 'bad epileptics or unclean paralytics' were admitted. This is one of the earliest observations of the tendency of central London hospitals partly to select patients to meet their own needs. This was to become more common as the teaching requirements of hospitals increased in the 20th century.

The hospital acquired a convalescent home in East Finchley and expanded both laterally and onto land behind the houses. In 1885 the houses were replaced with the red-brick building you see today. It continued to thrive and, in 1938, the Rockefeller Wing (the building to the right of the original hospital) was added. With the start of the NHS, it became the National Hospital of Nervous Diseases, and the University of London located the Institute of Neurology here. The hospital changed to its current name, recognising the surgical aspects of its services, in 1988.

Leave the square via Queen Anne's Walk (to the left of the hospital as you face it) past a modern

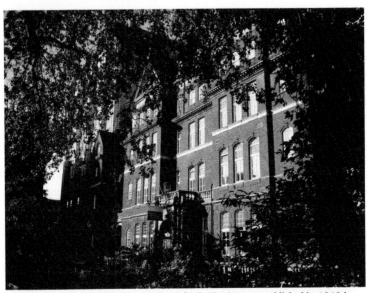

The National Hospital for the Paralysed & Epileptic was established in 1860 in houses on this site, which were replaced by this fine building in 1885. The Institute of Neurology's modern tower block can be seen beyond it

tower block, the main home of the **Institute of Neurology**. Turn right when you reach the road, Guilford Street. You are now walking along the northern edge of the Hospital for Sick Children. After about 50 m you pass the **Princess Royal Nurses Home** on your right, designed by Stanley Hall and opened in 1934. Despite its rather drab appearance, broken only by the bas-relief of Hygeia and other Greek gods over the entrance, it received an award from the Royal Institute of British Architects.

You then pass the Morgan Stanley Clinical Building that opened in 2012 and is the first part of the Mittal Children's Medical Centre, a multi-million pound redevelopment that will require the demolition of the Southwood Building that you saw earlier.

The next building is another postgraduate institute, the **Institute of Child Health**, established in 1947. After existing for nearly 20 years in borrowed space in the Hospital for Sick Children, this building opened in 1966. Stop when you reach the public drinking fountain, complete with steps to enable children to reach.

On the other side of Guilford Street is the entrance to the site of the former **Foundling Hospital**. The poor social conditions in London at the start of the 18th century meant that large numbers of children were abandoned, either orphaned or because their parents were simply not able to look after

Postgraduate institutes

Postgraduate education developed much later than that for undergraduates. Until the late 19th century, the need was largely met by the medical societies (p. 184). Four postgraduate institutes were established between 1893 and 1902. Despite these, when William Osler arrived from the USA in 1905 to be Regius Professor of Medicine at Oxford, he found that London was way behind cities such as Vienna. In 1911 he established the Postgraduate Medical Association, and after World War I the Fellowship of Medicine was set up to support doctors from the USA and British Dominions who had fought in Europe. In 1919 these two organisations merged, although they did not adopt a single name, the Fellowship of Postgraduate Medicine, until 1944.

Meanwhile, the Ministry of Health was developing its own plans, which culminated in the establishment of the Royal Postgraduate Medical School at the Hammersmith Hospital in 1935. At the end of World War II, the development of postgraduate education was finally taken seriously with the establishment of the British Postgraduate Medical Federation in 1947. It became a school of the federal University of London in 1951. At the same time, the royal colleges (p. 194) also started taking more responsibility.

While many hospitals created postgraduate education centres, the Federation established 14 specialist institutes in London, attached to appropriate hospitals (apart from the Hunterian Institute, which was based at the Royal College of Surgeons). The Federation, whose headquarters were in Bloomsbury (Gordon Square until 1955, and then Millman Street), survived until the 1990s, when it was dismantled, with the constituent institutes joining undergraduate medical schools.

them. Babies and young children left by their parents would starve and die in the streets in the most squalid circumstances. The only provision for them was the parish workhouses. In contrast, other European cities such as Rome, Venice, Vienna and St Petersburg had long-established orphanages and children's hospitals.

Appalled by the situation, Thomas Coram, a retired shipbuilder and sea captain, determined to establish a foundling hospital based on voluntary subscriptions. After an initial six years in temporary accommodation in Hatton Garden, a custom-built institution opened here in Lamb's Conduit Fields in 1745. At the time, this was the northern edge of the city, thus offering the children something of a rural idyll. A fine statue of Coram used to stand on top of the entrance.

The building was one of the most imposing monuments erected by 18th century benevolence. Designed by Theodore Jacobson, it consisted of a central block and two wings, one for boys and one for girls. Two colonnaded 'play sheds' connected

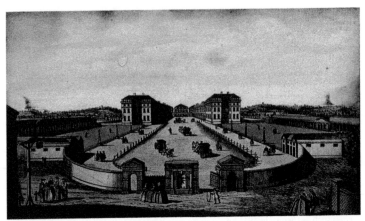

The Foundling Hospital, designed by Theodore Jacobson in 1745, was the first institution in London for abandoned infants. It closed in 1926, and all but the entrance and play sheds were demolished

the wings to the main entrance on Guilford Street which, as you can see, are the only parts of the original building that survive.

Foundlings were fostered with wet nurses in Kent and Surrey, returning to the hospital at five years of age to be educated and trained, often for domestic service (girls) or to be sailors (boys). In 1760 policy changed and unwanted illegitimate children from women 'of good character' were also considered for admission. However, as demand was high, infants were selected at random. Mothers were subjected to the anguish of having to draw a coloured ball from a bag to determine their child's fate: white meant admission (and giving up all rights to the child for ever), red meant the waiting list, and black meant rejection.

The Hospital created three valuable sources of income: a gallery (with work donated by Hogarth,

Reynolds and Gainsborough, which became the first public art gallery in Britain and led to the formation of the Royal Academy of Arts in 1768); a concert hall (Handel frequently performed *Messiah* here); and a chapel. Visitors were encouraged to attend Sunday morning services in the chapel and the concerts, following which they could view the paintings and the children. By all accounts, the girls were a more popular attraction than the boys.

By the 20th century, the site was no longer the rural idyll it had been in 1745. In addition, a plethora of other services, both statutory and voluntary, was available to support and care for vulnerable children and families. The Hospital closed in 1926, the main buildings were demolished, and the site was sold, although seven acres were preserved as the playground that you see before you. If you are accompanied by a child, you can enter the grounds.

Cross over Guilford Street and walk back in the direction you came. Turn right into Lansdowne Terrace, along the back of one of the playsheds, at the end of which is an entrance to Brunswick Square gardens. Walk through the gardens to the exit on the opposite side. The all-weather pitches on your right were the site of the main Foundling Hospital buildings. Leaving the gardens, you will see, to your right, a statue of Thomas Coram and The Foundling Museum (www.foundlingmuseum.org.uk), which contains the staircase from the boy's wing, the gallery and the court room from the original 18th century building.

In front of you to the left is the University of London's **School of Pharmacy**. Until the 1840s chemists and druggists were tradesmen or shopkeepers trained by apprenticeship, often fathers teaching their sons. The transition from these trades to that of pharmacists (p. 225) took a step forward in 1841 with the establishment of the Pharmaceutical Society of Great Britain. Formal training courses were set up not only by the Society, but also by several private schools. The transformation was formally recognised in the 1868 Pharmacy Act (ten years after the Medical Act regulating doctors), which enforced qualification by examination. This site was purchased for a new home for the Society, then based in Bloomsbury Square, but after years of deliberation and indecision only the School moved here (in 1949), while the Society later decamped to a new home in Lambeth.

Walk past the School of Pharmacy and turn right into Hunter Street. After about 50 m cross Hunter Street and stop on the corner with Handel Street. The building on the opposite corner used to be the **Royal Free Hospital School of Medicine**. Until the late 19th century, women were excluded from medicine. In this regard, Britain lagged behind other European countries. By the 1860s there were three female medical professors in Bologna, women were graduating in medicine from universities in Germany, and three women were studying medicine at the University of Paris.

The period 1866–76 was the decade of change in Britain. In 1866 Elizabeth Garrett, through perseverance and cleverly exploiting a loophole in the regulations of the Society of Apothecaries, managed to register as a doctor. Meanwhile, in 1869, Sophia Jex-Blake and six other women studied and passed the medical exams at Edinburgh, although they were denied a degree by the university. These revolutionaries joined forces with Elizabeth Blackwell, a British emigrant who had trained in medicine in the USA, to establish the London School of Medicine for Women. This was set up in a small house, The Pavilion, on this site in 1874. Two years later, parliament gave women the right to sit qualifying exams and to undertake clinical training in hospitals.

With public support from the likes of Charles Darwin and Lord Shaftesbury, the Royal Free Hospital,

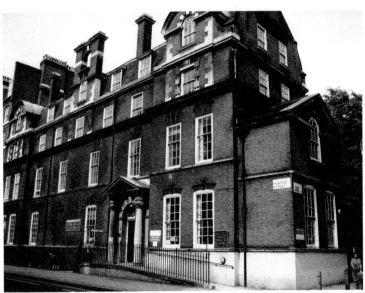

The former Royal Free Hospital School of Medicine, built in 1898 on the site of The Pavilion, the house in which its predecessor, the London School of Medicine for Women, had been established in 1874

true to its radical roots, cooperated. No other London hospital followed suit, and none of the other medical schools in London admitted women until 1916, when they were desperate for students, faced as they were with a shortage of men who had gone to fight on the front. By the late 1920s women were once again excluded (except at University College, where ten women a year continued to be allowed), and they were not readmitted until the medical schools were forced to do so, in 1947 to the University of London.

In 1898 the school was renamed the Royal Free Hospital School of Medicine. Demand from women wanting to train meant more space was needed, so The Pavilion was rebuilt and enlarged with the main entrance moved to Hunter Street. This is the building you see today. An additional wing, which completed the enclosure of the school's quadrangle, opened in 1916. Finally, another wing was added in Hunter Street in 1951, which you can see beyond the original building. The school moved, with the Royal Free Hospital, to Hampstead in the 1970s. Links with health care remain, however, as the Hunter Street building accommodates a health centre.

Carry on along Hunter Street to the junction with Tavistock Place. The red-brick building on the other side of Tavistock Place was where the **Central London Ophthalmic Hospital** moved to in 1925 when it left its original home, which you saw in Gray's Inn Road.

Walk 3

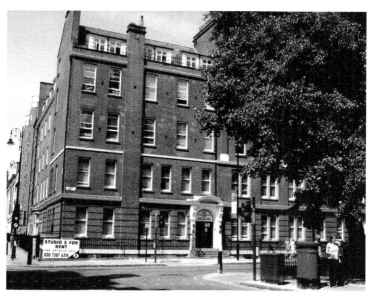

The Central London Ophthalmic Hospital moved from Gray's Inn Road to these purpose-built premises in 1925. Since the hospital left in 1988, the building has been converted into apartments

Despite many attempts to merge the three eye hospitals in central London, it was not until misfortune struck in the form of bomb damage to the Royal London Ophthalmic Hospital in City Road during World War II that any progress was made. Its outpatient department transferred here for a few weeks, long enough for the momentum for merger to build up. It finally happened in 1947. Clinical services were transferred from here to City Road, and this building was converted to house the Postgraduate Institute of Ophthalmology. It took until 1988 to unite all services plus the institute at City Road. The premises here are now private apartments.

Turn left along Tavistock Place and after 200 m turn left into Herbrand Street, where you will see, about 30 m on the right, the **Bloomsbury Ambulance Station**. Originally called Russell Square Station, it was one of only six built in 1915 when the London Ambulance Service was established by London County Council to deal with street accidents for the whole city. In 1930 the Service's responsibilities expanded to include the transport of sick (in particular, infectious) patients when it took over services run by the Metropolitan Asylums Board (p. 179). Ambulance staff became increasingly skilled in the immediate care of injuries and medical emergencies such that by 1974 the service became part of the NHS in order to facilitate greater integration with hospital care. It was then that this station was

Ambulances

Apart from some private ambulances to transport rich but infirm people in comfort that existed from the late 18th century, ambulances were introduced following a Parliamentary Select Committee recommendation in 1818 for a 'hospital carriage' for infectious patients so as to minimise the risk of spreading disease. In other words, it was more to do with protecting the public than with a concern for the person themselves. Initially, such carriages were hand-drawn litters, owned or hired by parishes and only adequate to convey patients short distances.

By 1879 the Metropolitan Asylums Board (p. 179) had instituted a city-wide system, with large fever hospitals outside London and a network of horse-drawn and river ambulances to transport fever patients to places of isolation, in particular Dartford. Six ambulance stations were established adjoining the hospitals, such that most of London was within three miles of a station. Each contained a house for the superintendent and house-keeper (a married couple), sleeping quarters for the staff, a kitchen, mess, stores, a coach-smith's forge, stabling for 15 horses, coach houses, omnibuses and an accident cart. An experienced nurse (summoned from the adjoining hospital) accompanied each carriage, together with a male assistant to help carry the patient.

Meanwhile, the increasing toll of industrial injuries in the rapidly expanding factories and dockyards led to a realisation of the need for first aid services. In 1877 the St John's Ambulance Association was formed by the Order of St John, heir to the Hospitallers, the religious order of knights formed in 1099 who were committed as much to nursing as to 'fighting the infidel'. The Association trained volunteers in first aid and nursing. By 1887 there were so many groups that the Order established the St John Ambulance Brigade to unite them all, and by 1912 there were 25,000 volunteers in the UK.

By 1900 the police in other cities were taking responsibility for transporting those injured in the streets. The City of London police introduced horse-drawn ambulance and hand litters, which they soon replaced with petrol vehicles and even an electrically driven ambulance, housed at St Bartholomew's Hospital. The service relied on 52 white telephone boxes in the streets. The rest of London had to wait until 1915, when the London County Council established the London Ambulance Service, consisting of six stations and 50 personnel. In 1930 it took on the responsibilities of the Metropolitan Asylums Board, acquiring an additional 150 petrol-driven ambulances and six large ambulances.

By 1948 there were 23 stations, 300 vehicles and 500 staff organised from a control room at County Hall. As ambulance staff became increasingly skilled in the immediate care of injuries and medical emergencies, and as mobile equipment became more sophisticated, it was apparent that ambulance services were an integral part of health care, the planning and management of which needed to be integrated with the rest of the health services. In 1965 the London Ambulance Service was combined with the eight other services covering the rest of Greater London, and in 1974 the combined service was transferred to the NHS. By 2006 there were 70 stations, 395 ambulances plus other paramedical services.

renamed. It is now one of 70 stations in London supporting nearly 400 ambulances (p. 106) plus other paramedical services.

Return to Tavistock Place, turn left, and at the traffic lights turn right into Tavistock Square. About 100 m on the right you will see Tavistock House, home of the **British Medical Association**. During the first half of the 19th century, many local organisations were established by doctors intent on 'maintaining the honour and respectability' of their profession, surrounded as they were by all manner of unlicensed practitioners. The latter they generally dismissed as charlatans and quacks. One of the more enterprising organisations was established in 1832 by Charles Hastings in Worcester, the Provincial Medical & Surgical Association. He saw the need for a united national organisation and,

Walk 3

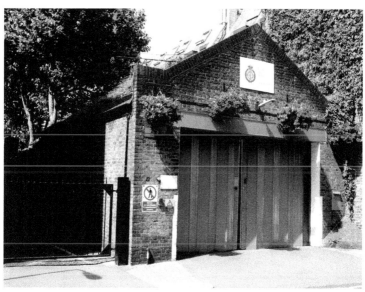

Russell Square Ambulance Station, one of only six established by London County Council in 1915 to deal with street accidents across the whole city

following several well-attended annual meetings, his association assumed that role. Renamed the British Medical Association (BMA) in 1856, the need for a London base if they were to influence policy became apparent.

Starting with two rooms in Holborn in 1871, the BMA expanded rapidly, necessitating frequent moves to increasingly large accommodation. The final move occurred in 1923 when it bought Tavistock House, which you can see across the courtyard beyond the ornate iron gates. It had been designed by Edwin Lutyens in 1913 for the Theosophical Society. At that time, access to Tavistock House was via a passage between two of the terrace houses that lined Tavistock Square.

The houses were demolished in 1938 and replaced with the buildings and entrance you are standing beside. Today, the BMA's concerns, as a trades union for doctors, are more to do with terms and conditions of employment than 'honour and respectability', although the difference may be less than it appears as their predecessors were largely motivated by their need to protect doctors' share of the health care market.

Leave the square along Upper Woburn Place, and after 70 m turn right into Woburn Walk (designed in 1822 as one of the first streets specifically for shopping). At the end, follow the old shop fronts round to the left and continue to Euston Road where, on the opposite corner, you will see the former home of

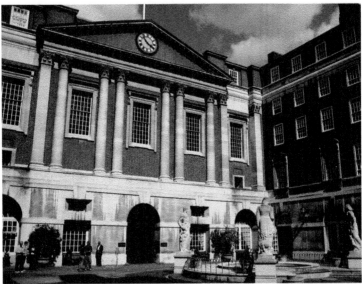

Tavistock House, designed in 1913 by Edwin Lutyens for the Theosophical Society, but instead, since 1923, it has been the headquarters of the British Medical Association

Walk 3

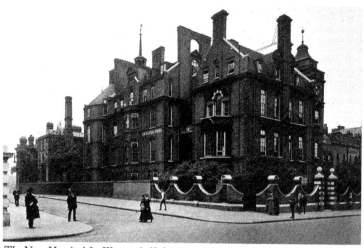

The New Hospital for Women, built in 1890, with its main entrance on Euston Road, was renamed the Elizabeth Garrett Anderson Hospital in 1917. It moved away in 2001, and part of the original building was preserved in the new UNISON headquarters (2011)

the **Elizabeth Garrett Anderson Hospital**.

In 1866, having registered as a medical practitioner, Elizabeth Garrett faced hostility from the male medical establishment. Unable to gain employment in any existing hospitals or dispensaries, she established St Mary's Dispensary for Women in Marylebone, staffed by women. It was renamed the New Hospital for Women in 1872 and moved to Marylebone Road, where 26 beds were provided. Exploiting another loophole, this time in the BMA's regulations, Garrett became a member in 1874, although her male colleagues moved quickly to ensure that she remained the only woman member of the BMA for almost 20 years.

The success of her hospital led to another move in 1890 to the custom-built premises you see on Euston Road today. The hospital, with 42 beds, aimed to be homely: central heating, polished parquet floors, open fires 'just to look at' and old brown milk jugs full of flowers. The original entrance on Euston Road can be seen. Following her death in 1917, the hospital was renamed the Elizabeth Garrett Anderson Hospital (she had married a Mr Anderson in 1893).

The founding ethos of the hospital was maintained when it joined the NHS in 1948. Indeed, the hospital had to gain exemption from the 1975 Sex Discrimination Act to continue its policy of female-only staff. Although it had grown to 161 beds, this was increasingly seen as being too small for a general hospital. So in 1979 it limited its work to gynaecology, in keeping with its original mission. However, the pressure for merger was unrelenting. In 1989 the Hospital for Women moved from Soho to share the building. Significantly, this brought male doctors onto the staff for the first time. Its geographical isolation still concerned people, and in 2001 it merged with the obstetric department of University College Hospital to form the Obstetrical & Elizabeth Garrett Anderson Hospital, originally in Huntley Street but now part of the new hospital in Gower Street.

Attempts to convert the abandoned building on Euston Road to meet the needs of a contemporary, disadvantaged group – drug addicts – were thwarted by opposition from local residents (supported by some women doctors) in scenes reminiscent of the reactions a few hundred metres away in 1763 when the residents of King's Cross opposed the foundation of the smallpox hospital. However, the building's connection with health care has been preserved. Although the magnificent circular wards at the rear of the site were demolished, most of the 19th century building has been beautifully restored and incorporated by the trades union UNISON, in its new national headquarters. Given that the union represents many low-paid women working in health care, part of the ethos of the building's original occupants lives on.

The walk ends here, near Euston underground station.

Walk 4: The challenging isle

Highlights

- first general hospital for women in London (Hospital for Women)
- first ENT hospital in London (Royal Ear Hospital)
- only specialist hospital in London for men with venereal disease (London Lock Hospital)
- first and most famous private anatomy school (Great Windmill Street School)
- second general dispensary to be established in London (Westminster General Dispensary)
- leading skin hospital in Britain (St John's Hospital)
- largest dental hospital in Britain (Royal Dental Hospital)
- first home of Charing Cross Hospital
- home of the Royal College of Physicians for 136 years

Start: Tottenham Court Road underground station
Finish: Piccadilly Circus or Charing Cross underground station
Length: 2.9 km (1.5 hours)

At the heart of the great metropolis lies an island, a foreign land in a sea of Englishness. Since its development in the 17th century, Soho has always been different from the villages and districts that surround it. It has challenged and threatened the rest of London while, at the same time,

enticing and nourishing it. The reasons are bound up with its origins.

Until the 1660s this was hunting country. Development so close to the City was forbidden for fear of contagious diseases spreading to within the City walls. However, when the Great Fire of 1666 left 100,000 homeless such a policy had to be abandoned as refugees flocked west in search of new beginnings. Despite the fact that Soho was born out of an urgent necessity, it rapidly became a fashionable area. Development started in the south with Old Compton Street and Golden Square in the 1670s, and then spread north via Dean Street and Wardour Street to Soho Square in the 1680s. Property was bought by wealthy city merchants wanting to be closer to the royal palaces of Whitehall, Westminster and St James. By 1700 there were 60–80 titled residents, 27 MPs and many foreign ambassadors and envoys here.

Meanwhile, the first of a succession of waves of refugees seeking sanctuary, tolerance and opportunities arrived. Following the revocation of the Edict of Nantes in 1685, about 15,000 Huguenots fleeing religious persecution arrived from France, such that by 1711, 40% of the parish was French. The air of freedom and non-Englishness created by the politicised Huguenots encouraged natives of other countries to settle here as it was seen as being an area where alien

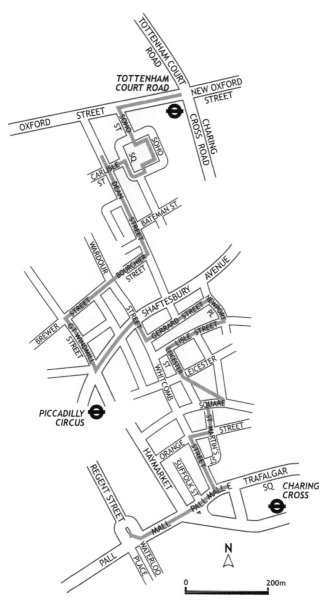

traditions would be tolerated and accepted.

By the mid-1700s the nobility and gentry started to shift further west to Mayfair and beyond. They were partly replaced, in the 1760s, by Greeks escaping persecution from Turkish occupiers, and in the 1790s by more French, this time fleeing from the terror that their own revolution unleashed. Little wonder the area was still referred to as 'petty France' in the 1840s. And still more foreigners arrived: political refugees from Germany and from Italy following failed revolutions in the 1840s; Russian and Polish Jews escaping the pogroms of the 1880s. By 1900 Soho must have been one of the most cosmopolitan urban areas in the world, for in addition there were Swiss, Belgians, Swedes, Austrians, Dutch, Spaniards, Hungarians, Danes and Americans. Later, from the 1920s onwards, they were joined by Chinese migrants.

The new arrivals may have had little wealth to contribute but they brought with them their food, their art and their energy to create the vibrant and convivial atmosphere that Soho has always had. This in turn attracted the unorthodox, the non-establishment, the difficult – artists, revolutionaries, writers and musicians. Marx, Casanova, Canaletto, Marat, Hogarth, Blake, De Quincey, Dryden, Garibaldi, Mozart … And with artistic and intellectual freedom came sexual liberalism. Alongside its reputation for international food and dining, from 1800 Soho became notorious for night clubs, erotic shows and prostitution, fuelled by a ready supply of impoverished residents in areas to the east, St Giles and Covent Garden, desperate for work.

While men of the governing classes in their West End homes were happy to enjoy the informality of what was on offer in the brothels and molly-houses of Soho, they wanted the area contained. In 1816–24, in a

rare act of the Crown using its power to transform the city, 700 properties were swept away in order to create Regent Street, a boundary between the nobility of Mayfair and the riff-raff of Soho. (Even then, the colonnaded arcades in the grand new street, built to allow the upper class to shop in all weathers, had to be demolished as it was felt they encouraged prostitutes.)

An unintended but lasting benefit of such overt social engineering has been that Soho is the best preserved area of London (helped by the lack of bomb damage during World War II). Its street pattern has hardly altered in 300 years. Buildings of domestic simplicity on a human scale have survived, with few high-rise developments. It remains an island, a foreign land entered from Oxford Street to the north, Charing Cross Road to the east, Regent Street to the west and Leicester Square to the south. The contrast between Mayfair and Soho has persisted and can still be felt today on crossing Regent Street. For over 200 years Soho has offered visitors informality and excitement, be it food from all corners of the world, entertainment or sex.

The enduring character of Soho has inevitably shaped the health services that have developed or been attracted here. The atmosphere has encouraged individuality, creativity and entrepreneurship, the main theme of this walk. Soho is somewhere to take risks, to challenge orthodoxy. The departure of the nobility in the mid-1700s provided the opportunity for members of the newly established professions (including medical practitioners) to move in and establish commercial and charitable enterprises:

John Hunter, who transformed surgery; his brother, William, who established the first anatomy school; George Armstrong, who established the first dispensary for sick children in England; and John Lind, who founded what was only the second general dispensary in London. They were followed in the 19th century by John Harrison Curtis, a naval surgeon with no formal medical qualifications, who established the first ear hospital in England, and Benjamin Golding, a young doctor who established what was to become Charing Cross Hospital.

The second theme of this walk arises from the consequences of sexual liberalism. Venereal disease, the 'Foul Disease', had been ever-present in all social strata of London. With the exception of the Middlesex Hospital (from 1803) and the Royal Free Hospital (from 1828), general hospitals refused admission, fearing contagion. However, by 1850 realisation of the need for services to meet this challenge resulted in the establishment of no less than three specialist hospitals in Soho that openly treated venereal diseases: after nine years in Red Lion Square, Protheroe Smith moved what was the first hospital exclusively for 'diseases of women' to Soho Square; the first hospital in London for men with venereal diseases, the Lock Hospital, was established in Dean Street; and John Laws Milton set up St John's Hospital for skin diseases, many of which would have been venereal in origin. Additional services, particularly for female prostitutes, were provided by another Soho institution, the Hôpital et Dispensaire Français.

The third theme of this walk is the way medical entrepreneurship has driven change in health care. In addition to establishing specialist hospitals, medical practitioners (and surgeons in particular) set up private anatomy schools. From the moment the surgeons separated from the barbers in 1745 to create their own City company, schools or theatres of anatomy were established in which corpses were dissected. By 1836 there were 21 in London, three of them in Soho, including the first and most prestigious, in Great Windmill Street.

The social character of Soho and the key theme of the walk is well illustrated by two towering figures in the history of health care, one of whom you will encounter at the start and the other at the end. Shortly after entering 'the isle', you will see the home of Mary Seacole, daughter of a freed black Jamaican slave who, although rejected by the authorities, went and nursed wounded British soldiers on the battlefield in the Crimean War. She personified Soho – relaxed, openly loving with a *joie de vivre*. Later, as you reach the southern and western shores of Soho, you return to the establishment world, the former homes of the Royal Dental Hospital and the Royal College of Physicians. And there, amid the gentlemen's clubs of St James's, a grand monument to the Crimean War complete with a fine statue of Florence Nightingale, the daughter of wealthy middle-class parents but, in contrast to Seacole, anguished and emotionally retentive. The bas-reliefs on the monument show nurses tending the injured. But there is no sign of 'Mother Seacole'.

The walk starts at Tottenham Court Road underground station. Leave the station via Exit 1. On emerging, turn left along Oxford Street and after about 150 m enter Soho by taking the first left, Soho Street. This brings you into Soho Square. Cross over and enter the gardens. Turn left and stop after 10 m, opposite No. 14.

Soho Square, originally known as King's Square, was laid out in 1681. All the original houses have been replaced so the square is now a hotch-potch of buildings from different periods, many of them lacking any architectural charm. Although recently refurbished, No. 14 dates from the early 19th century. For three years, this was the home of a pioneering figure in British nursing, **Mary Seacole**. Born in Jamaica in 1805, her mother was a freed black slave and her father a Scottish army officer. Having learnt nursing skills from her mother, Mary voluntarily went and cared for the victims of a cholera epidemic in Panama (after the doctor had fled the scene). Her devotion to British servicemen brought her to London to offer her services to the government to go and nurse the injured in the Crimean War. After several rejections, she raised her own funds and set up a nursing home, the British Hotel, in 1855 near Balaclava to provide 'a mess-table and comfortable quarters for sick and convalescent officers'. Unlike Florence Nightingale, who was stationed 300 miles away across the Black Sea in Scutari, 'Mother Seacole', as she was known, nursed the wounded on the battlefield.

She returned to London, destitute and in ill-health. With the help of well-wishers, she cleared her debts and, in 1857, came to live on the fourth floor of 14 Soho Square, a boarding house. Belatedly, she gained some recognition from the establishment, although Nightingale dismissed her as a 'brothel-keeping quack'. Despite this, she was hugely popular with the public, as reflected in the 80,000 people who attended a grand military festival in her honour at the Royal Surrey Gardens. In 1860 she returned to Jamaica but came back in 1870 and lived out her life in west London, dying in 1881.

Walk on round the gardens and stop opposite No. 22, a rather unsympathetic recent addition. This was the site of the **Dispensary for the Infant Poor**, the first dispensary for sick children in England. It was established by George Armstrong (along with seven other Scottish doctors) in 1769 at a time when up to half the infants of the poor died and many physicians believed nothing could be done about it. The dispensary was initially located in Red Lion Square but moved here in 1772. Armstrong, who had published one of the first textbooks on children's diseases, encouraged prevention through cleanliness, breast-feeding and warmth, in addition to treatment. The dispensary saw poor children for free on three days of the week, although the landlord required them to enter by the back door. On three other days of the week, private patients were seen, admitted via the front door.

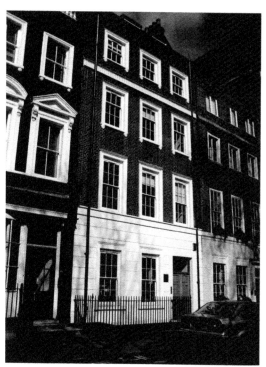

For three years, Mary Seacole lived in rooms on the fourth floor of this house after returning from nursing injured troops in Crimea

Despite providing free treatment to the destitute, Armstrong was not immune from criticism, perhaps because he had trained and qualified in Scotland and was not licensed by the Royal College of Physicians of London. Even one of the most enlightened reforming physicians of the day, John Coakley Lettsom, was opposed to Armstrong's unique work, claiming that 'lives are being sacrificed to experimental mass treatment'. Sadly, Armstrong ran out of funds, despite spending half his time seeing private paying patients. He was committed to a debtor's prison and, after his release, died

unrecognised in 1789. And as if that weren't bad enough, even after his death he was denigrated while at the same time his published work was plagiarised. It was not until the 20th century that he finally gained the recognition he deserved. The dispensary was, arguably, the most important step ever taken in England towards the care of sick children.

Carry on round to the next gateway where an information board gives you an idea of how the square looked when first built. Leave the gardens and walk 10 m to the right so you are opposite **The Hospital for**

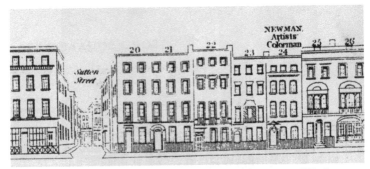

Established by George Armstrong and seven other Scottish doctors, 22 Soho Square housed the first dispensary for children in England from 1772 until its demise in 1781

Women. Established by Dr Protheroe Smith in 1842 in Red Lion Square as the Hospital for Diseases of Women, it aimed to treat 'those maladies which neither rank, wealth, nor character can avert from the female sex'. It was soon renamed because the title, with its association at the time with venereal diseases (p. 123), put off potential supporters. It moved here in 1852, initially occupying one house, but a decade later the neighbouring house was acquired and the two were rebuilt with two extra storeys. Like all voluntary specialist hospitals (p. 119), it depended on a variety of charitable sources. It was fortunate in benefiting from the proceeds of the week-long Soho Fair & Market held in the square every year. Among the stalls and attractions were the intriguingly named 'Smokey Cohen's' and 'The Electrical Association for Women'. In addition to charity, from 1879 it attracted 'a superior grade of sufferer who are able to pay for their own support', suggesting that the understandable fears and concerns that middle- and upper-class women might have had about hospitalisation

had been overcome thanks to the hospital's fine reputation. The hospital's success can also be gauged by further expansion behind the building, along Frith Street.

The façade you see today was added in 1910. Despite the pressure on specialist hospitals to merge or to become part of a large general hospital, it remained independent, even after its incorporation into the NHS. However, it succumbed in 1989, when its services were transferred to the Elizabeth Garrett Anderson Hospital on Euston Road. Subsequent mergers and moves mean that Protheroe Smith's institution is now lost in the obstetric and gynaecology department of Elizabeth Garrett Anderson & Obstetric Hospital, part of the modern University College Hospital in Gower Street.

The building here in Soho Square still provides health care. It houses general practices, dentistry, support for the homeless and drug addicts, as well as a centre for the local Chinese community and, since 2000, the first NHS Walk-in Centre.

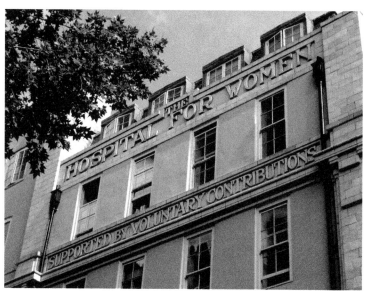

The Hospital for Women, established in 1842, moved into two houses in Soho Square in 1852, and the houses were enveloped in this façade in 1910

Walk 4

Voluntary specialist hospitals

The establishment of voluntary specialist hospitals challenged the social order in medicine. The first tranche, established in the middle of the 18th century, specialised in conditions excluded from the general hospitals (pregnancy, contagious diseases, skin diseases, insanity, venereal disease). The second tranche, in the 19th century, focused either on specific organs – eyes, ears, 'chest', heart – or on groups who were not made to feel welcome in many general hospitals – women, children and foreigners.

Unlike voluntary general hospitals (p. 148), specialist hospitals were usually established by an entrepreneurial doctor, reacting to the conservatism of powerful medical interests. Opportunities for career advancement in general hospitals were limited to the families, friends and favoured pupils of the established doctors. Those not so privileged, dissatisfied with their prospects and sufficiently entrepreneurial could try to establish a specialist institution.

The secret of success was the ability to attract financial support and the involvement of some well-known doctors. The founder needed to cultivate friends in commerce, trade and industry to become subscribers, for whom the incentives were similar to those for subscribers to general hospitals, although often the 'rewards' did not extend to influence over admissions, appointments and terms of service.

Given their origins, it was no surprise that specialist hospitals attracted considerable criticism. General practitioners, who were competing for patients and income, and voluntary general hospitals, which competed for charitable donations and good teaching cases, were vehemently opposed (although many general hospital doctors could not resist also holding an appointment at a rival specialist hospital). The medical establishment (dominated by the general hospital doctors) challenged the knowledge and skills of the doctors in the specialist hospitals, who, it was claimed, made unjustified claims for greater knowledge and skills. Such 'medical upstarts' were felt to be principally concerned with self-promotion and self-advancement. But they could not just be ignored because they diverted good teaching cases away from general hospitals.

Apart from criticism from peers, specialist hospitals faced the same abuses of their charity as general

hospitals by those who could afford to pay a private practitioner and by subscribers in effect using them as a means of providing medical insurance for their employees and servants at a cheap rate. In addition, general hospitals started creating their own specialist departments (causing the governors of some specialist hospitals to ban their doctors from also holding posts in general hospitals). Like general hospitals, some specialist hospitals established convalescent homes to clear 'bed blockers'.

Despite opposition from much of the medical establishment, by 1869 there were 64 specialist hospitals in London, with an average of 73 beds each, alongside 11 general hospitals with almost 400 beds each. Inevitably, funding voluntary hospitals (p. 159) could be precarious, and many small specialist hospitals were short-lived. However, some survived, played a leading role in the development of their specialty, and are now world-famous institutions. The NHS adopted the main ones in London as regional or national centres, handling difficult, rare and unusual cases.

Continue on to the corner of the square. Across the road, you can see the entrance to Twentieth Century House, which continues round the corner, occupying what was No. 32. Until its demolition in the 1930s, No. 32 was an 18th century building similar in appearance to No. 26, which you came past on the opposite side of the square. If you

look back you can see the elongated fan light extending over the door and side windows. The house at No. 32 was, if anything, more spectacular than its surviving mirror image. It was also of considerable historical importance, having been Joseph Banks' home, which was in effect the centre of British botany and home of the Linnean Society (the world's

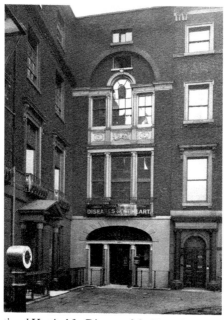

Home to the National Hospital for Diseases of the Heart from 1874 to 1914; a box outside the entrance, with the plea 'Spare one penny', requested donations

oldest extant biological society) until the 1850s. Following this illustrious history, it served as the original home of the **Dental Hospital of London** and the **London School of Dental Surgery** from 1859 until 1874. After they moved to Leicester Square, the house was taken over by another, well-established specialist hospital, the **National Hospital for Diseases of the Heart**. This was the third home for what was the first hospital in the world specialising in cardiovascular disease. It remained here until 1914 when it moved to custom-built premises in Marylebone.

Cross over and leave the square by Carlisle Street. Note the porticoed entrance to No. 38 on the opposite side of the street. It was here, in

1816, that John Harrison Curtis established the first ENT hospital (p. 82) in London, the **Dispensary for Diseases of the Ear**, which was to prove as controversial as it was successful. He was viewed by licensed doctors as a notorious quack as he had no recognised medical qualifications. However, much to their frustration, he had married a woman of considerable means and social connections, resulting in him coming to the attention of royalty and the aristocracy.

Within four years the dispensary's popularity meant it needed more space. If you continue along Carlisle Street, you can see the site (although not the building) of the dispensary's second home on

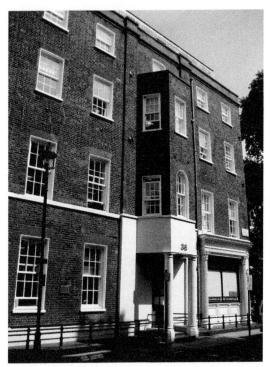

The first home, from 1816 to 1820, of the Dispensary for Diseases of the Ear, the first ENT hospital in London, which was to become the Royal Ear Hospital

the corner with Dean Street (now a pizza restaurant). By 1820 Curtis had become aurist to George IV and other members of the royal family, making him immune to the diatribes launched by fellow practitioners. In 1822 George IV became patron of the dispensary, which became known as the Royal Dispensary for Diseases of the Ear. This served to incense further the physicians and surgeons of the royal colleges. The dispensary, which remained on this site for 56 years, will be encountered again later on this walk.

Meanwhile, turn right into Dean Street and stop after 20 m opposite

the entrance of an extensive, neo-Georgian, stone and red-brick building. As you can see from the notice carved in stone over the door, this was the Male Hospital, a branch of the **London Lock Hospital** that had been established by William Broomfeild (sic) in 1746 in Grosvenor Place, behind Buckingham Palace gardens. The main hospital served both men and women with venereal disease who were excluded from the general hospitals because they were deemed to have sinned. It aimed both to cure the body and to reform the patient's morals. For the latter, an asylum to rehabilitate female patients was established in Paddington, where women spent up to two years being reformed and trained for domestic service. A similar facility for male patients was not deemed to be necessary. Alongside the main hospital in Belgravia, an 800-seat chapel was built, which, thanks to popular preachers, provided a third of the income from the rent for pews. It was arranged so the patients could not be seen by the rest of the congregation. The fame of the chapel was compromised when in 1780 one preacher, Martin Madan, advocated polygamy as a solution to prostitution.

By 1842 the hospital was no longer welcome as Belgravia was becoming fashionable with the nobility. Both the hospital and the chapel moved to Paddington, where they were united with their asylum as the London Lock Hospital &

Rescue Home. While the new location provided a God-fearing congregation and a retreat from the city, it was inaccessible to those most in need. So in 1862 a branch opened here in Dean Street in an 18th century townhouse for outpatients and male inpatients. This coincided with the period of the controversial Contagious Diseases Acts (1864–86) that allowed for the compulsory detention of any women whom the police believed were prostitutes. The hospital, which benefited greatly from government funding to meet the requirements of the Acts, had to expand at both its sites to meet the demand.

Despite the fall in income following the repeal of the legislation, the hospital was rebuilt in 1912. This is the building you see today, designed by Alfred Saxon Snell. It had 33 beds on the upper floors and urethral irrigation

Walk 4

Venereal disease

Until 1740 the only hospital care for those with venereal disease were the 'foul wards' at St Thomas' Hospital and two former leprosy hospitals. In 1746 the first voluntary specialist hospital (p. 119) in London (of any kind), the London Lock Hospital, was established well outside the city, in Grosvenor Place. The name probably derived from the Old French, *loques*, meaning rags, and referred to the dressings that patients wore to cover their sores. To meet patients' spiritual needs, the Lock Hospital built a large chapel (which also

proved to be a useful source of income as it rented out the pews) and in 1792 established an asylum (or rescue home) in Paddington where female patients could repent and 'abandon the primrose path that leads to the everlasting bonfire'.

While wealthy men could pay private surgeons to treat them at home, there were few services available for the less affluent: two voluntary general hospitals started to provide treatment in the early 19th century (Middlesex Hospital in 1807, Royal Free Hospital in 1828), and there were the newly established skin hospitals (p. 132), which did not, or could not, distinguish venereal from other causes.

In the 1860s politicians saw venereal disease as a threat to the security of the country. They felt that male soldiers had to be protected from female prostitutes by, under the 1864 Contagious Diseases Act, requiring 'prostitutes' in garrison towns to undergo compulsory examination and, if deemed infected, inpatient care for up to three months. Enacting the policy meant no woman was safe from being detained at the say-so of the local police. The Ladies Association, led by Josephine Butler and Elisabeth Wolstenholme, opposed what they saw as a harsh, sexist policy. However, the Act was supported by The Lancet, the British Medical Journal (from 1867) and Elizabeth Garrett Anderson, who felt it offered protection and help to impoverished women. Meanwhile, the Lock Hospital benefited from generous government funding. However, opposition persisted and the Act was repealed in 1886.

The importance of venereal disease in men had been recognised by the establishment of a branch of the Lock Hospital for men in Soho in 1862. The only other facility to be established was a small hospital 'For Skin & Genito-Urinary Diseases' founded by Dr Felix Vinrace in 1897. Recognition of the military importance of venereal disease in men was heightened during World War I and led to a second period of government funding (from the War Office). After the war, the Metropolitan Asylums Board (p. 179) established the Institution for Venereal Diseases, near Lincoln's Inn Fields, for women (which was renamed Sheffield Street Hospital in 1930) and St Margaret's Hospital in Kentish Town for infants born with ophthalmia neonatorum. London County Council also started funding St Paul's Hospital (the new name for the hospital founded by Vinrace), much to the chagrin of the Lock Hospital, which was struggling financially.

The advent of sulphonamides and then antibiotics in the 1940s and 50s led to the premature judgement that venereal disease could be eliminated and therefore specialist services would no longer be needed. Primary care and the genito-urinary medicine departments of general hospitals were left to cope as the specialist hospitals closed.

cubicles on the ground floor where men came for their daily treatment delivered by nurse orderlies including the appropriately named Messrs Rodwell, Hardstand and Catchpole. The hospital enjoyed a second period of prosperity during World War I when the government responded to the threat that venereal disease posed to the health of its fighting force. Demand for treatment increased, particularly in Soho as the area attracted servicemen from many nations on leave. Government funding had to be kept secret through fear of hostility over the use of public money for this purpose.

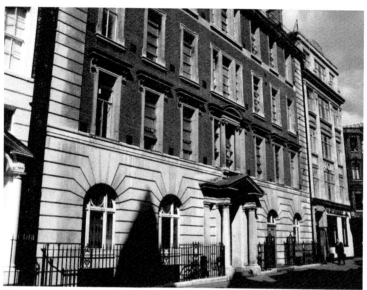

*The London Lock Hospital's male branch, designed by Alfred Saxon Snell in 1912,
which survived until 1952. Sadly, it has now been abandoned and is awaiting a
new use*

Following the war, the hospital struggled financially because other institutions were preferred by the Metropolitan Asylums Board (p. 179) and its successor, the London County Council. In addition, policy was shifting from specialist to general hospitals. Finally, the advent of new drugs – sulphonamides and then penicillin – led people to believe that venereal diseases were soon to disappear. The Lock Hospital for men was incorporated into the NHS in 1948, but within four years it had been closed.

An additional reason for the closure was the need for a new home for the **West End Hospital for Neurology & Neurosurgery**, whose buildings in Marylebone and Regent's Park had suffered bomb damage in 1940. Established in 1878, this was the only specialist hospital for diseases of the nervous system apart from the National Hospital in Queen Square. It took over the old Lock Hospital building here in Dean Street in 1952 and remained until 1972. Long before roof terraces became fashionable in central London, the matron, Mrs Welch, established a roof-top garden for the benefit of staff and patients. In 2012 the building remained largely abandoned, although a primary care centre was occupying some of the ground floor.

Turn and walk down Dean Street (away from Oxford Street). About 50 m on the right is St Anne's Court. The modern building on Dean Street just beyond was the site of several houses, one of which housed St James' & St Anne's Dispensary from 1858 to 1880, a general dispensary for the working poor. Continue for about 100 m and stop on the corner with Bateman Street. No. 72 (Royalty House) on the opposite side of Dean Street occupies the site where, in the late 18th century, the Dean Street School of Anatomy was established. This was one of at least 21 private anatomy schools (p. 128) that existed at the time. It survived until 1830, when it moved to become, in effect, Westminster Hospital Medical School.

The house in Dean Street on the other side of Bateman Street has a blue plaque in recognition of Dr Joseph Rogers, an apothecary and surgeon, who lived there from 1821 to 1889. Rogers, together with Louisa Twining and Charles Dickens, led the reform of the workhouses. In 1866, while working as the medical officer at the **Cleveland Street Workhouse** in Fitzrovia, he established the Association for the Improvement of London Workhouse Infirmaries, which led to the establishment of 20 new public hospitals, with professional nursing, for the poor. His obituary in the *British Medical Journal* referred to him as the 'Hercules of workhouse reform'.

Cross Dean Street and continue along it until you reach Bouchier Street. 42–43 Dean Street, on the opposite side, was where the **Royal Dispensary for Diseases of the Ear** moved to in 1904. Pride in being the oldest ENT hospital in London

is apparent from the prominence given to its foundation date, which adorns the façade in gold lettering. Despite the passage of time, other aurists (ear doctors) in London still resented the special place that the 'Royal Dispensary' occupied. The King's response was to incense them further by referring to it as The Royal Ear Hospital. By the early 20th century, support for all small specialist hospitals was waning. Mergers or amalgamations with a general hospital were seen to be the alternative ways forward. The Royal Ear Hospital opted for the latter and in 1920 amalgamated with University College Hospital, although it did not move to its large, purpose-built premises in Huntley Street, near to its parent hospital, for another six years. Its old premises now house a restaurant on the ground floor and part of the private members' Groucho Club on the upper floors.

Turn down Bourchier Street; at the end, cross Wardour Street and continue along Brewer Street. Take the second on the left, Great Windmill Street. About 100 m on the left, immediately after the Windmill Theatre, is a red-painted brick façade with a blue plaque. You can see it better from the other side of the road. This is all that remains of the first and most famous private anatomy school in London, the **Great Windmill Street School**. The school was established by William Hunter, a Scottish surgeon, within months of the Company of Barber-Surgeons splitting in 1745. Until then the only places where dissection of the human body were permitted were the Barber-Surgeons' Hall and the Royal College of Physicians. Hunter offered students the opportunity to study anatomy using the French or Parisian method (where sophisticated schools had existed for at least 25 years), a euphemism for dissection of a human corpse.

For 22 years the school was based in houses in Covent Garden and the Haymarket, and for much of that time William Hunter was assisted by his younger brother, John. In 1768 William Hunter commissioned a purpose-built school, the façade of which you see today. Designed by Robert Mylne, it included an anatomy theatre and a museum to house his thousands of anatomical preparations covering the whole animal kingdom. The façade has been altered over the years – there used to be a central entrance with a classical portico. Some of the ground- and first-floor windows with 12 panes of glass remain (as in the second bay from the left), as do all the smaller top-floor windows.

The school was immensely popular, with 100 students often

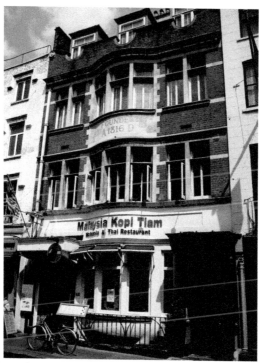

The third home, from 1904 to 1926, of the Royal Ear Hospital, which proudly displayed in gold lettering, between the first- and second-floor bay windows, the year it had been established

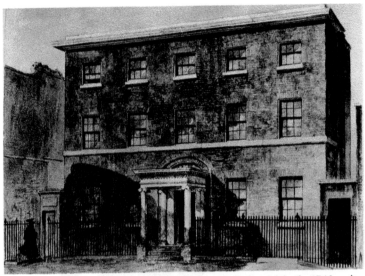

The Great Windmill School of Anatomy, designed by Robert Mylne in 1768, as it looked in its heyday when it was the leading theatre of anatomy in London

Private anatomy schools

Until the surgeons broke away from the barbers in 1745, anatomical demonstrations were only permitted at the Barber-Surgeons' Hall and the Royal College of Physicians. The new freedom to teach anatomy was first exploited by William Hunter when he established a school in 1746. However, it was not until 1769 that the first purpose-built private school opened in Great Windmill Street (at least 25 years after similar schools in Paris). Many others followed, mostly established by Hunter's acolytes, such as Great Queen Street School (1777) by John Sheldon, Blenheim Street School of Anatomy (1787) by Joshua Brookes, Webb Street Theatre of Anatomy (1819)

by Edward Grainger, and Little Windmill Street School of Medicine (1822) by George Dermott.

By 1836, 21 private schools existed. Most included a theatre in which dissections could be observed and a museum for studying specimens. Lecturers were physicians and surgeons at the nearby voluntary hospitals. Courses in anatomy were held in the winter months when bodies did not decay so quickly. However, in 1787 Joshua Brookes discovered how to preserve bodies by embalming, which allowed dissection in the summer months.

The demand for an anatomical education was not confined to

doctors – according to the *Medical Times*, 'a knowledge of anatomy was then very properly considered a necessary accomplishment to a gentleman and indispensable to the lawyer.' Advertisements made no mention of dissection, instead referring to 'teaching in the French manner' or 'practical anatomy'. The demand for corpses for dissection encouraged resurrectionists (grave-robbers). One of the more horrific consequences occurred to John Sheldon in 1784 when his sister's body was delivered to him.

Towards the end of the 18th century, three of the large voluntary general hospitals (p. 148) started their own medical schools: the London in 1785, followed by St Bartholomew's and St Thomas' & Guy's. Teaching was largely oriented to surgery, which, in turn, was limited to externally obvious conditions (such as abscesses and fractures) as knowledge of 'internal' medicine was still scant.

The growing demand for bodies for dissection (there were 1,000 students in London each year) could not be met from those executed and this led not only to grave-robbing but also to people being murdered and their bodies sold.

The 1832 Anatomy Act abolished the law that limited dissection to criminals' corpses, thereby removing the stigma of leaving your body to a medical school. In addition, schools and teachers had to be licensed and the remains had to be properly buried. As a result, the supply of bodies rose.

By the 1840s most voluntary general hospitals had their own school, sometimes by assimilating one of the private ones. Although one private school survived until 1914 (Cooke's in Brunswick Square), the rest had closed by the 1860s.

Walk 4

present. While dissecting the corpses of hanged criminals was legal, the activity remained controversial and students were discouraged from discussing what they saw and heard with members of the public. Guests were permitted to attend most lectures, although not those 'on the organs of generation and the gravid uterus'. The audiences were not restricted to aspiring surgeons. At the time, knowledge of anatomy was 'very properly considered a necessary accomplishment to a gentleman and indispensable to the lawyer'.

The demand for corpses for dissection encouraged resurrectionists (grave-robbers) whose activities had horrendous consequences. In 1784 John Sheldon of the Great Queen Street School was horrified when his sister's body was delivered to him. The anatomists' demand for bodies, particularly young healthy bodies, and the prices they were prepared to pay led to people being murdered. While Edinburgh had Burke and Hare, London had Bishop and Williams.

The importance of the Great Windmill Street School was

immense as many of the other schools were set up by pupils of Hunter. The school continued to prosper after Hunter's death in 1783 despite him bequeathing the entire contents of his museum to Glasgow University. However, by the 1830s the voluntary general hospitals (p. 148) had established their own medical schools, partly because education was shifting from the dissection room to the wards, and partly because it was a lucrative activity. The days of the private schools were drawing to an end. This one closed in 1836, and the building became a French restaurant before being incorporated into the Lyric Theatre in 1887.

Walk on and turn left onto Shaftesbury Avenue. Take the second on the right, Wardour Street, and then second left, Gerrard Street. About 100 m on the left is No. 9, with a strange porticoed double entrance. This building started life in 1759 as the Turk's Head pub, a favourite of Samuel Johnson, Joshua Reynolds and others who, in 1764, founded The Literary Club here. Following the closure of the pub in 1783, it was home to the Linnean Society until 1821. Meanwhile, the **Westminster General Dispensary** had been established nearby in 1774, only the second general dispensary (p. 229) to be established in London, the first having been set up in Aldersgate four years earlier. In 1825, in need of more space, it took over this building. Although the building is largely unchanged, it had a more elegant stucco finish in the 19th century as well as the name of the dispensary emblazoned across

the façade. The dispensary flourished here for over a century and, despite the availability of free primary care (p. 211) under the NHS, it continued due to public demand until 1956.

Continue along Gerrard Street, turn right into Newport Place and then first right into Lisle Street. Cross over and walk about 100 m until you reach Leicester Place. To meet the needs of the large French-speaking population of Soho, a French doctor, Achille Vintras, established a dispensary in 1861 in Charlotte Street, north of Oxford Street. The need for a hospital was soon apparent so, in 1867, the dispensary moved and expanded to become the Hôpital et Dispensaire Français in a house in Lisle Street, on the site of the present-day Prince Charles cinema (beside you). It remained here until 1889, when it moved to custom-built premises at the top end of Shaftesbury Avenue.

Carry on along Lisle Street and stop when you reach Leicester Street. The somewhat incongruous building on the other side of Lisle Street (No. 5), built in a new renaissance style with a big stepped gable and crowned by an obelisk, was designed by Frank Verity in 1897 for The French Club. Later it became the London headquarters for Pathé of France before being acquired in 1935 by **St John's Hospital for Diseases of the Skin**, a specialist skin hospital that had been established 72 years earlier.

During the 19th century, the public (and most practitioners) made little distinction between skin diseases. All were assumed to be contagious, and sufferers were

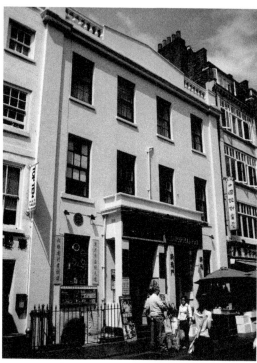

Now a Chinese supermarket, this was home to the Westminster General Dispensary for 131 years from 1825, during which time its name was emblazoned on the stuccoed pediment

stigmatised and excluded from most voluntary general hospitals (often in the belief that the cause was venereal in origin). Some specialist skin hospitals (p. 132) and dispensaries were created, although by 1860 there were still only three. In response, in 1863, John Laws Milton, a surgeon, together with three other doctors, established St John's Hospital in a house near Great Compton Street. From the start, the institution was dogged by disputes. Within a week, Milton's three colleagues had resigned as they objected to him associating

the new hospital with a publication on spermatorrhoea (involuntary ejaculation). The view that it was a malady that needed treating was, at best, controversial in medical circles. This, however, did not stop Milton running a highly lucrative clinic to 'treat' it.

Despite this setback, the hospital survived and moved to a large house in Leicester Square in 1865 (long since demolished). However, although the need for treating skin diseases was great, the topic did not easily attract subscribers and donations, forcing the hospital to

Walk 4

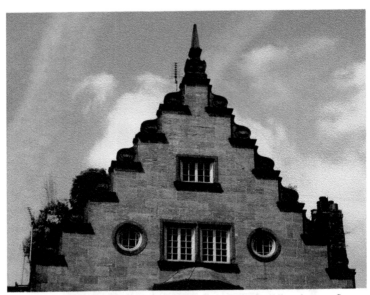

The big stepped gable of Frank Verity's 1897 French Club building, home to St John's Hospital for Diseases of the Skin from 1935 to 1990

Skin hospitals

In medieval times, little distinction was made between different skin conditions, including leprosy (p. 17). All carried the same stigma. As a result, many of the patients in leprosy hospitals may have been suffering from other conditions. After the demise of those hospitals in the 16th century, there was no institutional provision for those suffering from skin conditions (apart from the Lock Hospital for women with venereal disease (p. 123)) until the late 18th century. At that time, some of the physicians and surgeons working in the first voluntary dispensaries, such as Robert Willan and Thomas Bateman, developed a special interest in skin diseases.

As the voluntary general hospitals tended to exclude such patients, specialist dispensaries and hospitals developed. The first in London was the London & Westminster Infirmary for the Treatment of Diseases of the Skin in Great Marlborough Street in 1819. No more appeared until the London Infirmary for Diseases of the Skin in Great Ormond Street in 1835, but over the following 22 years seven more were established, including the Hospital for Diseases of the Skin in 1841. It was founded by James

Startin at London Wall as the London Cutaneous Infirmary but soon moved to Blackfriars, where it remained until 1948. It was to become the leading skin hospital in the UK for 70–80 years.

Eventually, the general hospitals accepted skin conditions, starting with University College Hospital in 1859. Charing Cross Hospital did so a year later, but it took until 1908 for all the large voluntary hospitals to recognise the importance of skin conditions. Meanwhile, six more specialist hospitals had been created, including, in 1863, St John's Hospital. Despite being dogged by controversy (due to the personality of the founder, John Milton Laws), from the 1920s it replaced the hospital at Blackfriars as the premier skin institution.

Until 1948 dermatology had a close association with venereology due to the large number of skin conditions attributable to an underlying venereal disease. Some specialist hospitals, such as St Paul's Hospital in Covent Garden, had to decide which path to pursue.

The development of dermatology was helped by the establishment, in 1882, of the Dermatological Society of London. Membership was restricted to 60 and was by invitation only. *The Lancet* felt that it was extremely influential, 'bringing order out of chaos'. In 1895 a rival medical society (p. 184), the Dermatological Society of Great Britain & Ireland, was founded. However, the small size of the dermatological community precluded the viability of two organisations so they merged in 1907 and affiliated with the Royal Society of Medicine. To promote the interests of those doctors specialising in skin conditions, the British Association of Dermatologists was founded in 1920. While the specialty has prospered, skin hospitals gradually closed during the 20th century. The last was St John's Hospital, which merged with St Thomas' Hospital in 1990.

Walk 4

abandon its charitable principles and give priority to patients who could pay. Some funds were also raised through teaching, which by 1885 led to the creation of a school of dermatology. Soon after, however, two incidents once again disrupted the life of the hospital: the matron and nurses resigned when Milton ignored professional roles and instructed a cook to do a dressing; and an inquiry was held into financial irregularities.

The hospital survived for 70 years in Leicester Square before moving here in 1935. The hospital's claim to be the premier skin hospital in London was endorsed in 1946 when the University of London located one of its postgraduate institutes (p. 101) here. An expansion of clinical services into properties behind the hospital in Gerrard Street followed. However, like other small specialist hospitals, the pressure to merge was great, and in 1990 St John's Hospital, together with the Institute, moved to St Thomas' Hospital.

Walk down Leicester Street and into the garden in the centre of Leicester Square. Ever since the 18th century, the square has been the focus of exhibitions and spectacles. These used to include health care, such as that put on by James Graham in the 18th century, whose celebrated displays of medicinal mud-bathing were aided by 'a bevy of belles'. Walk diagonally across the gardens to the far corner, where you will see a badly weathered bust of **John Hunter**, the founder of modern surgery. The reason for it being placed here is that, from 1783 until his death in 1793, he lived nearby at No. 28. His house was replaced in 1897 by the six-storey building you see today.

John Hunter, younger brother of William, arrived in London in 1748 at the age of 20 having received little education. Assisting William in his anatomy school, he immediately revealed an extraordinary talent for dissection and anatomy. He went on to train in surgery, spending three years abroad as an army surgeon. He returned to London in 1763, settled in Golden Square, Soho and developed a successful private practice. This enabled him to purchase land in Earl's Court, build a house and pursue his fascination with comparative anatomy by establishing a menagerie of living animals including leopards, ostriches and jackals.

One of his clinical interests, which developed as an army surgeon, was venereal disease. At the time, the distinction between syphilis and the less serious gonorrhoea was not recognised. The notion of protection through inoculation was enticing given what had been achieved with

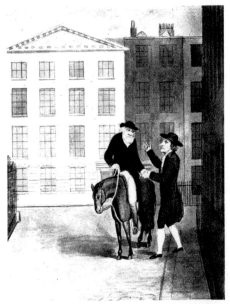

In 1783 John Hunter shows his new house in Leicester Square to a friend

smallpox since the 1720s. In 1767 Hunter tested the idea by introducing the infected discharge from a female prostitute into the penis using a lancet! He may even have subjected himself to this and, as result, contracted syphilis, which might explain his long-delayed marriage and his later ill-health. Needless to say, the idea did not catch on.

By 1783 his fame and wealth allowed him to buy not only 28 Leicester Square but also the house behind it. He then commissioned a vast museum, 52 feet long, to be constructed between them. Like his brother, he was accumulating a huge collection of anatomical specimens from across the animal kingdom. As many as 29 people worked for him, including resident pupils. His desire to expand his collection extended to bribing undertakers to supply the body of an Irish fairground giant. Following his death in 1793, the collection of 14,000 specimens (including the giant) was bought by the government and given to the Company of Surgeons. It can be visited at the Royal College of Surgeons in Lincoln's Inn Fields (www.rcseng.ac.uk/museums).

Leave the gardens and you will see to your right the imposing Hampshire Hotel, which occupies half the south side of the square. This was built in 1901 as the **Royal Dental Hospital**, which had started life as the Dental Hospital of London in Soho Square. It had first moved in 1874 to two houses that stood on the site of the Odeon cinema, which can be seen to the right of the hotel. The decision to

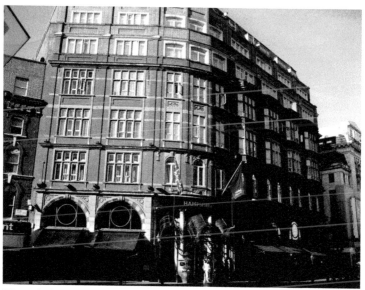

The majestic Royal Dental Hospital, built in 1901, with shops at ground level as an extra source of income. After the hospital left in 1985, it was converted into a hotel

Walk 4

move there was controversial as, at the time, the square was 'overgrown with rank and fetid vegetation ... and an unwholesome fever-bed'. Although the hospital was a success, demand and activity were such that, by 1898, the Dean of the dental school described the accommodation as 'insanitary and unsavoury'.

Rather than rebuild on the existing site, the adjacent site was acquired. Development was nearly prevented by members of the temperance movement who were campaigning against the sale and consumption of alcohol (p. 136). Their concern was that

the collection of buildings on the new site included a pub that, along with other existing shops, would be accommodated in the ground floor of the new hospital as a source of income. They felt that a hospital dependent on income from a pub was a 'scandalous proposal'. Despite this, construction went ahead, but as the pub survived for only two years, in the end all parties gained satisfaction. Shop fronts still line the street today, with the one furthest to the right still in use. On moving into the new building in 1901, the hospital gained its Royal prefix.

Alcohol

Until the mid-19th century, high levels of consumption of alcoholic drinks were understandable given the lack of clean water (p. 259). However, concern about its harmful effects led in 1835 to the foundation in Preston of the British Association for the Promotion of Temperance. At its peak, 10% of the population had joined the temperance movement and taken a pledge to abstain from alcohol. Temperance halls were built to hold meetings to extol the virtues of abstinence and provide education and entertainment. The movement sought to close down pubs or convert them into temperance hotels or coffee houses.

A particular challenge was the key role of alcohol in medical treatment, which was curiously specific: port was prescribed for patients undergoing a tracheostomy,

brandy for cancer of the throat, stout for ulceration of the trachea, champagne for a partial laryngectomy, and brandy and whisky for typhus. Hospitals often spent as much on alcohol as on nursing or on other drugs. Given the lack of anaesthetic agents before the 1850s, alcohol probably provided a welcome escape for those undergoing surgery. Larger hospitals even employed their own brewer on the premises. And alcohol was not only provided for patients. Two-thirds of expenditure in one workhouse infirmary was for alcohol consumed by staff. Not surprisingly, staff drunkenness was a major problem. In response, in 1873, the temperance movement founded the London Temperance Hospital, which discouraged (but did not outlaw) the prescribing of alcohol.

The hospital provided only outpatient care, the few patients requiring admission being housed in nearby Charing Cross Hospital until the start of the NHS in 1948. Almost as soon as the hospital was incorporated into the NHS, and despite the opposition of the staff, a new home for the hospital and the school outside central London was sought. However, despite several attempts, it took almost 40 years for a move to take place. Finally, in 1985, the dental school was merged into the United Medical & Dental Schools (Guy's & St Thomas'). However, the dentists preferred to see the hospital's clinical services dispersed rather than be forced to move en masse from central London.

All mention of its history is omitted from the hotel's publicity, perhaps sensing the apprehension guests may feel about sleeping with the ghosts of dental drills.

Walk down the right-hand side of the hotel (St Martin's Street), first right (Orange Street) and then left down Whitcomb Street. At the end, on Pall Mall East, you are opposite one of the former homes of the **Royal College of Physicians,** now part of Canada House.

The westward movement of medical practitioners in the early 19th century, in pursuit of the nobility and gentry who paid for private care, was accompanied by the two royal colleges (p. 194). The surgeons set up home in Lincoln's Inn Fields in 1813, where they have

Walk 4

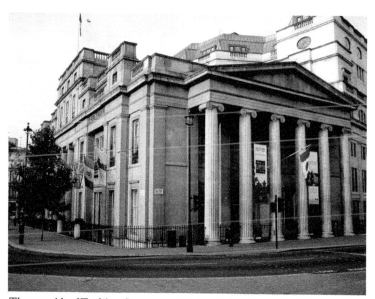

The west side of Trafalgar Square, developed by Robert Smirke in 1827, provided a neo-classical home for the Royal College of Physicians until 1963 (foreground) and a home for the Union Club (beyond)

stayed to the present day, while the physicians moved here in 1827. The neo-classical building, with six mighty Doric columns, was designed by Robert Smirke. Its severity may have suited the College's grandees, but even at the time it was felt to be 'severe almost to the point of dullness'. In 1875, the façade was lightened somewhat by the addition of statues of Linacre, Harvey and Sydenham in the three niches behind the columns (later removed).

If you look down the left-hand side of the building you will see how it was part of a larger edifice occupying the west side of Trafalgar Square. The other half was built for the Union Club, a gentlemen's institution, which in 1923 they sold

to the Canadian High Commission. When the physicians left their part in 1963 (to move to Regent's Park), the High Commission expanded and united the two.

Walk away from Trafalgar Square along Pall Mall East and stop after about 30 m on the corner of Suffolk Street. At the top of this short street, you can see it is closed off by an impressive four-storey, late-18th century house to which an extra storey was later added. In 1818 a young, idealistic doctor, who was increasingly concerned about the lack of medical care available for the poor and deprived, established the **West London Infirmary & Dispensary** in the building. In 1825 Benjamin Golding moved

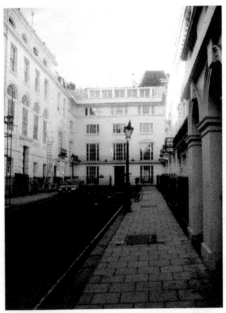

The West London Infirmary & Dispensary (which became Charing Cross Hospital) was established in the 18th century house across the end of the street

his hospital to Villiers Street, off the Strand, and two years later it acquired its permanent name, Charing Cross Hospital.

Continue along Pall Mall East, cross Haymarket and walk on until you reach Waterloo Place. Cross to the Crimean War Memorial on the traffic island. Erected in 1915, about 60 years after the war, it is unique among war memorials for commemorating not only the servicemen who lost their lives, but in addition the contribution of nurses, one in particular – **Florence Nightingale**. While this partly reflects the decisive contribution that Nightingale made at the time and subsequently in civilian life, it may also serve to distract attention from the otherwise incompetent execution of the war by the leading soldiers and politicians involved.

The magnificent bronze statue of Nightingale stands on an ornate pedestal bearing four bas-reliefs illustrating her diverse roles: caring for the injured; negotiating with politicians and generals; challenging medical and hospital managers; acting as a teacher and inspiration to nurses. Forever remembered as the Lady of the Lamp, Nightingale played a key role in the 19th

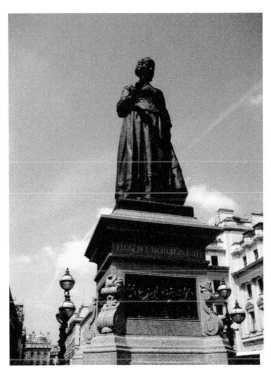

The statue of Florence Nightingale erected in 1915 to commemorate her contribution to the Crimean War some 60 years earlier

Walk 4

century transformation of nursing from an occupation of disrepute to the modern profession it has become. Her key contributions were the reform of army medical services, improving hospital design, establishing nursing education, developing statistical monitoring of performance, and advising on sanitary reform in India. She was one of the great reformers of health care.

It is appropriate that her statue stands here near the heart of power where the establishment has worked and played for generations. For Nightingale was only able to achieve so much because of her own social position and the access that gave her to government ministers, generals, aristocracy and other influential people. But unlike other women with such opportunities, she used them to bring about profound change. Ironically, in her determination and commitment to relieve the suffering of the ill and injured, she probably had more in common with a self-taught nurse from Jamaica who on returning from the Crimean War resided in a cheap boarding house in Soho, less than a mile away, but in many ways, on a foreign island in the sea of London.

The walk ends here a few minutes from Charing Cross and Piccadilly Circus underground stations.

Walk 5: Merge or move

In the 1750s London extended only as far north as Oxford Street. Beyond lay fields and orchards. The Tottenham Court Fair, held near the site of present-day Warren Street underground station, included such attractions as bear-baiting, bull-baiting and women boxers. However, with the construction of the New Road in 1756 (renamed Euston Road in 1857) linking Paddington and Islington, London started to grow such that by 1830 the land between Oxford Street and New Road had been laid out in terraces and squares, including such architectural gems as Fitzroy Square and Bedford Square.

The area bounded by Gower Street to the east and Great Portland Street to the west became known as North Soho. Initially, it was a fashionable residential area, but later in the 19th century the wealthy started moving west to Mayfair and Belgravia. Some of the vacated houses were turned into workshops, mainly for furniture-making, a tradition that is still evident from the furniture stores on Tottenham Court Road. Other houses were divided into cheap flats, attracting less affluent, more bohemian residents, particularly painters and writers. By the 1930s the Fitzroy Tavern in Charlotte Street had become the nerve centre of the louche local scene. Those frequenting it became known as Fitzrovians and the area acquired the name by which it is known today, Fitzrovia.

While some commentators have characterised this area on the basis of its artistic community, the area also serves to illustrate a key feature of the evolution of health services: the tendency of dispersed facilities to join together, creating ever-larger institutions. During the 20th century, most of the hospitals established in Fitzrovia during the 18th and 19th centuries repeatedly merged, culminating at the start of the 21st century with a single solitary giant at

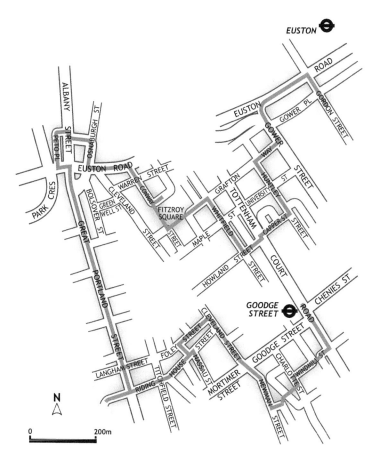

the north end of Gower Street, rising high over the district. This is the result of a final 'showdown' between the last two major players, the Middlesex Hospital and University College Hospital.

The power of this centripetal force extended outside the local environs as small hospitals to the south of Oxford Street and north of Euston Road also got sucked in. The Middlesex Hospital attracted the Central London Sick Asylum, Arthur Stanley Institute for

Rheumatology, part of the Royal National Orthopaedic Hospital, and four urology hospitals. Meanwhile University College Hospital collected the National Dental Hospital, the Royal Ear Hospital, the Hospital for Tropical Diseases, the National Temperance Hospital, the Elizabeth Garrett Anderson Hospital, the Hospital for Women, and the Heart Hospital. And finally these two hospital giants merged.

While aggregation has been a powerful influence on the

development of hospitals, it has not been all-powerful. Some smaller establishments pursued another option. A centrifugal force led them to move away from central London to less crowded and less expensive areas that provided opportunities for expansion: Mount Vernon Hospital outpatients joined its inpatients in Northwood, part of the Royal National Orthopaedic Hospital moved to Stanmore, the Metropolitan Ear Nose & Throat Hospital went to Kensington, St Saviour's Hospital went as far as Hythe in Sussex, and the London Foot Hospital moved to Stratford in east London.

A second influence on the development of health services that can be vividly seen in this part of London is religion. University College, formed by dissenters and free-thinkers opposed to the Anglican dominance of Oxford and Cambridge universities, was forced to establish its own hospital to provide clinical training for its medical students as they were excluded from the Middlesex Hospital. The latter viewed the 'godless institution in Gower Street' as an inappropriate partner. This was at a time when it was compulsory in Middlesex Hospital for all staff and ambulant patients to attend the weekly religious service in the hospital boardroom.

Close links between health care and religion took several forms. The transformation of nursing and, as a result, the salvation of hospitals was led by religious sisterhoods in the second half of the 19th century, the most famous being St John's House based in Fitzrovia. Even atheistic

University College Hospital resorted to the All Saints Sisterhood in 1862 to modernise its services. Other local manifestations of the influence of religion were the establishment by Catholic sisters of St Saviour's Hospital in 1873; the creation of the London Temperance Hospital, encouraged and supported by a movement that often took the form of a religious revival with 'baptisms' and 'excommunications'; and the establishment of a hospital exclusively for the Anglican clergy, St Luke's in Fitzroy Square.

A third theme is the emergence of paying patients. Up until the 1880s hospitals were generally dangerous places for inpatients. Health care had little to offer in the way of effective treatments, and there were risks of acquiring additional infectious diseases. Only those with poor home conditions and no alternative access to care made use of them. Reorganisation of hospital care, largely led by nurses, changed the views of the middle classes. It was here in Fitzrovia that the impact of such changes was first seen. In 1878 the first hospital in the UK exclusively for paying patients, Fitzroy House, was established. This was partly a consequence of most voluntary hospitals refusing to allow paying patients, although by the end of the 19th century financial pressures led them to change their policy and establish pay-beds. Later they went even further and built 'private wings': the Middlesex Hospital succumbed in 1929 and University College Hospital in 1937.

Philanthropy is the fourth theme. Voluntary hospitals depended on the generosity of individual donations for capital developments. Although early examples exist – Samuel Whitbread, the brewer, provided a cancer ward at the Middlesex Hospital in 1791 – philanthropy was largely a 20th century activity. At the Middlesex Hospital, John Astor (whose wealth came from hotels) provided a nurses' home; James Buchanan (whiskey), a private patients' wing; Henry Barnato (diamonds and breweries), a cancer institute; Edward Meyerstein (novelist), a radiotherapy institute; Edmund Davis (diamonds and banking), murals in the entrance hall; Samuel Courtauld (textiles), an institute of biochemistry; Thomas Ferens (cleaning materials), an institute of otolaryngology; Jules Thorn (electric lighting), an institute for clinical science; Daniel Ludwig (shipping), a cancer research institute; William Morris (cars), an institute of nuclear medicine; and Isaac Wolfson (retailing), a psychiatry department. Meanwhile, at University College Hospital, the Rockefeller Foundation (oil) provided an obstetric hospital, doctors' residences and a nurses' home, Donald Currie (shipping) paid for the medical school and a nurses' home, John Maple (furniture) funded a whole hospital, Max Rayne (property) a research institute, Joseph Duveen (art dealer) the Royal Ear Hospital, and Isaac Wolfson (retailing) a medical research institute.

A fifth theme is the ill-defined and changing distinction between accepted, orthodox medicine and alternative, non-orthodox practices and practitioners. Some therapies currently available from non-orthodox practitioners used to be accepted by orthodox medicine: phrenology was championed by one of the first professors of medicine at University College in the 1830s, until he and his beliefs were hounded out of medicine; colonic irrigation 'to purge the body of toxins', so favoured today by some, was a mainstay of treatment in rheumatology clinics in the 1930s and 40s; and electro-homeopathy, recently enjoying a renaissance, was widely practised at St Saviour's Hospital for Cancer in the late 19th century. Conversely, some practices have travelled in the other direction: the Middlesex Hospital was the first hospital in London to establish an electrical department and make use of electrotherapy, previously the province of non-orthodox practitioners.

Finally, there has been a long-standing interest in the development and provision of cancer care in Fitzrovia. The cancer ward established at the Middlesex Hospital in 1791 was the first in the UK. Cancer remained a particular interest of the hospital – it was the first to undertake experimental treatments using radioactivity soon after Marie Curie's discovery in 1897. Meanwhile St Saviour's Hospital provided palliative care, Mount Vernon Hospital shifted its interest from TB to cancer in the 1930s, establishing a radium institute in Riding House Street, and St Margaret's Clinic for Tumours was established in 1935 on Euston Road.

This walk, which begins with a hospital established in two small terraced houses in 1745 and ends with a 17-storey tower opened in 2005, illustrates the way hospitals have developed not only in London but in cities throughout the world.

Walk 5

The walk starts at Goodge Street underground station. On leaving the station, turn right along Tottenham Court Road. In 1750 this was the main route out of London to the distant village of Highgate. The only buildings at the time were a row of houses, long since demolished, on your right. This was a rural area for farming and recreation. After 150 m turn right at the Rising Sun pub into Windmill Street and stop after about 50 m opposite No. 8, all that remains of the original **Middlesex Hospital**. The rest of the hospital, Nos 9 and 10, have been rebuilt.

Apart from the 'royal' hospitals of St Bartholomew's, St Thomas' and St Mary Bethlehem, established in the 12th and 13th centuries, the first voluntary hospital in London was the French Huguenot Hospital, which opened in 1718. The following 30 years saw five more established – Westminster, Guy's, St George's, the London and, in 1745, Middlesex Hospital. It was to be 75 years before another emerged.

Initially based in two terraced houses (Nos 8 and 9), the Middlesex Infirmary for the Sick & the Lame of Soho expanded in 1747 to occupy a third (No. 10). Among the medical staff was the renowned William Hunter, who was not only a surgeon but also one of the newly emerging man-midwives (obstetricians). His involvement guaranteed a place in history for the Middlesex Hospital as the first general hospital in England to include childbirth (p. 22). However, the high demand for 'lying-in', which often meant two to a bed, threatened the availability of beds

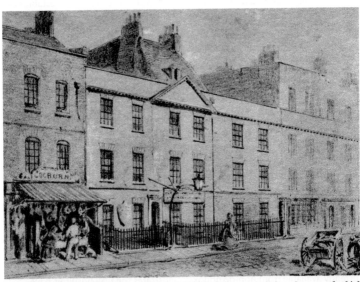

The first home of the Middlesex Hospital (1745–57) occupied three houses, of which only the right-hand house, No. 8, has survived. Patients were chastised for hanging out of the windows to chat with passers-by

for other purposes. Despite half the hospital's 40 beds being allocated to lying-in, the man-midwives' appetite for expansion could not be met. So after a few years they left to set up the first specialist lying-in hospital in England. Despite their departure, the governors' desire to expand persisted and led them to seek a new site for a purpose-built hospital. In 1754 they found one, just a few hundred metres away in Marylebone Fields, known at the time as 'a good place for snipe shooting'.

Little is known about these houses in Windmill Street after the hospital left in 1757 apart from a 13-year period from 1839. No. 10 is famous in the history of dentistry (p. 187) as the home of the first dental hospital and school in the UK, the **London Institution for Diseases of the Teeth**.

Walk on along Windmill Street to the corner with Charlotte Street, where you will see on your right the Fitzroy Tavern, the hostelry that gave the area its name. In 1750 you would have seen, on the opposite side of Windmill Street, the **Middlesex County Hospital**, the first infectious diseases hospital (p. 78) in London established to provide care for sufferers of smallpox. It accommodated only 13 patients, which after a few years proved insufficient. It moved, in 1753, to a much larger purpose-built hospital in Coldbath Fields (modern-day Mount Pleasant) and was renamed the London Smallpox Hospital. On the other side of Charlotte Street, No. 21A housed the Western Dispensary for Diseases of the Skin from 1856 to 1866.

Cross Charlotte Street, go through Percy Passage, cross Rathbone Street and through Newman Passage continuing until you reach Newman Street. These streets give you an idea of the area in the 19th century. Turn right and after 100 m you will reach Goodge Street.

From 1757 until 2005 you would have been gazing upon one of London's major hospitals, the Middlesex Hospital, which occupied the site to the left on the other side of the road. All that remains is the hospital chapel, which, in 2012, is preserved in the centre of a wasteland awaiting redevelopment.

Despite attracting generous donations for developing its buildings, like other voluntary general hospitals (p. 148) it struggled financially with running costs. In 1788 only four of the 16 wards were open. This was exacerbated after 1793 with the economic downturn resulting from the Napoleonic wars. The governors sought both to cut costs and to increase income. Despite its charitable status, the hospital raised funds by admitting paying patients when the opportunity arose, such as when French clerics driven into exile by the revolution offered to pay. To reduce costs, the food rations of the resident staff were reduced and savings were also made in treatment costs: linseed meal was substituted for bread in the poultices; the doctors' use of the newest, and therefore most expensive, medicines was curbed; and the leeches used, which had risen to 100 a day (these being imported from France), had to be preserved and reused.

Walk 5

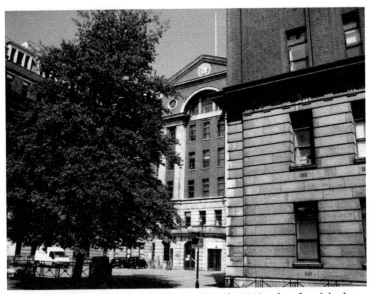

The former Middlesex Hospital building, built in the 1930s when the original 18th century building was in danger of collapsing. It was vacated in 2006 and demolished in 2010

Voluntary general hospitals

In 1718 in St Luke's parish, French Huguenots established a hospital for sick and infirm fellow refugees based on the French custom of hospitals being funded by better-off citizens. This was to serve as a model for the way hospitals were created, financed and governed for the next 200 years in England. Eighteenth century London, with its new prosperous middle class and the increasing influence of non-conformists (such as Quakers), was receptive to the new approach. Within a year, groups of concerned citizens had established Westminster Hospital, followed by St George's (1733), the London (1740) and the Middlesex

Hospital (1745). More were to follow in a second flurry of activity in the 19th century, including Charing Cross (1818), Royal Free (1828), University College (1833) and King's College Hospital (1839). This second tranche was as much to meet the needs of students and teachers as the needs of patients.

The key means of funding voluntary hospitals (p. 159) was subscriptions. There were several motives to become a subscriber:

- religious – to demonstrate religious devotion and to find favour after death

- philanthropic – from a benevolent concern about the well-being of others
- social pressure – the risk of ostracism if not seen to be contributing
- self-advancement – the opportunity to make useful business connections, particularly for members of the middle class to meet the upper classes
- efficiency – (mis)use as cheap health insurance for employees (including domestic staff)
- profit – subscribers were favoured when contracts for hospital supplies were placed.

Although voluntary hospitals greatly enhanced the opportunity of hospital care for a large proportion of the population, the working poor still needed a subscriber's letter of recommendation, could only be admitted as inpatients on certain days of the week, sometimes required proof of funds to pay for their own funeral (hardly encouraging) and often had to supply their own linen, cutlery and food.

Voluntary hospitals had their critics. First, there were suggestions that such charity did more harm than good by engendering dependency and irresponsibility. Second, they were said to have unfairly diverted business from private doctors, threatening their income. There was also conflict between doctors and governors over who selected the patients for admission. Governors were concerned that the financial benefits the doctors received in tuition fees (directly from students) might lead them to prioritise patients who best met their teaching needs. They challenged doctors' control further in the 1890s when Lady Almoners (p. 85) were introduced in outpatient departments partly to ensure that free care was not being abused by those who could afford to pay. Governors also sought control over medical appointments in a bid to challenge what they saw as a nepotistic and corrupt system.

Despite the introduction of a variety of funding mechanisms to supplement voluntary subscriptions, expenditure always exceeded income, and hospitals struggled from one financial crisis to the next. Despite protestations by hospitals, incorporation in the NHS in 1948 meant they finally reached safer shores where their future, even if not guaranteed, could be planned and managed.

Walk 5

Another source of income was medical students. In the 1820s, when the main source of students, the private anatomy school (p. 128) in Great Windmill Street in Soho, started to decline in prestige, an obvious alternative was University College, established in 1828, which needed a hospital for its medical students. But the college was non-conformist, something abhorrent to the high-minded Anglican governors of the Middlesex Hospital, who rejected any connection with 'the godless institution in Gower Street' and created their own medical school in 1835. It was to be over 150 years before the two big beasts of north London would settle their differences and merge.

Cross over and walk 100 m down Cleveland Street, to the right of the old hospital site, as far as No. 44, a four-storey brick building on the right, behind a scooped brick wall. Its simplicity and lack of decoration belie its historic importance. For this, the **Cleveland Street Workhouse**, is the last remaining Georgian workhouse in London, which continuously served the health care needs of Londoners for over 230 years (until 2005). The central building with protruding lateral wings (one for men, one for women) was built in 1778 by St Paul's parish in Covent Garden as their workhouse. This was probably the workhouse that influenced the young Charles Dickens, who, from 1829, lived for several years at No. 22 (in a house you just passed). During the 1850s and 60s it was the focal point for the leading social reformers of the day, most notably Dr Joseph Rogers, the 'Hercules of workhouse reform' who served as medical officer for the workhouse, and Louisa Twining, who created the Workhouse Visiting Society. Their work resulted in National Inquiries and eventually an Act of Parliament that was to transform the lives of the impoverished and infirm throughout the country.

In 1829 St Paul's was merged with neighbouring parishes to form the Strand Poor Law Union, with this building becoming the Workhouse Infirmary. In 1870 the Union was combined with other unions, by the recently established Metropolitan Asylums Board (p. 179), to form the Central London Sick Asylum District. The Board had ambitious plans to build six infirmaries in London, but funds only allowed two to be constructed, one of which was achieved by extending the existing buildings here such that there were 264 beds, similar in size to its neighbour, the Middlesex Hospital.

With the end of the Board in 1930, the building was acquired by the Middlesex Hospital and converted to house its outpatient clinics and ENT department. The latter transferred to the Royal National Throat, Nose & Ear Hospital in 1997, and the outpatients went to the new University College Hospital in 2005. In 2011, following a campaign, the historic and architectural importance of the Georgian workhouse building was recognised when it was listed, ensuring it is preserved within any redevelopment of the site.

Cross the street and walk down Foley Street. About 50 m on the right is the entrance to **John Astor House**. Built in 1931, this nurses' home (p. 151), paid for by Lord Astor, sought to meet (or maybe create) the needs of the residents. It included a swimming pool, recreation room, reading room, hairdressing salon, garden, tennis court, badminton court and, curiously, a photographic darkroom. On the left side of the street, the School of Pathology and School of Radiography were constructed. Continue to the corner of Candover Street and look back towards John Astor House. You will

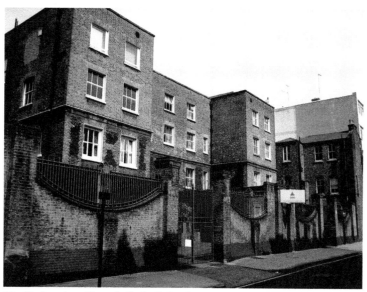

The H-shaped workhouse built for St Paul's parish in the 1770s later formed the centre of a workhouse infirmary for the Strand Poor Law Union (1829) and then for the Central London Sick Asylum (1870). In 2012 it awaits redevelopment

see, attached to it, the **Macdonald–Buchanan Nursing School**, added in 1959. Like all hospital nursing schools, it closed in the 1990s when its responsibilities were transferred to a university.

Nurses' homes

Until the 1850s hospital nurses' status resembled that of servants. They were expected to sleep in the wards or in the garrets. The introduction of nursing sisterhoods (p. 163) transformed not only nurses' work, but also their hours, pay, food and accommodation. Initially, nurses were still accommodated within the hospital, but from about 1870 nearby houses were acquired.

Some small purpose-built nurses' homes were introduced in the 1900s, but most were not built until 1925–35 (often with philanthropists' donations) to meet the rapidly expanding needs of the hospitals. As living in was a requirement, hospitals with insufficient accommodation encountered difficulties staffing their wards. The hierarchical nature of the nursing profession was reflected in the arrangements in these vast new buildings. Sisters, staff nurses and probationers were carefully segregated,

Walk 5

and their accommodation reflected their status. Each group had its own sitting room, and the best appointed homes included reading rooms and sports and other facilities.

Changes in social conditions and attitudes meant that, by the 1950s, the compulsory requirement for nurses to live in was threatening the ability to retain staff. In 1953 the Ministry of Health recommended that living in was only necessary for matrons, acute ward sisters and first-year nursing students. From the government's point of view, they could relinquish the responsibility for building and maintaining so many homes, although the reasons espoused were the greater independence it gave nurses and that closer contact with the outside world would instil greater insight into the problems faced by patients.

Turn left into Candover Street. At the end, cross over into Nassau Street. You are now on the west side of the former main hospital site. Walk halfway down the right-hand side of the street. Two buildings (shrouded in scaffolding in 2012 because all that remains are their façades) here illustrate the hospital's involvement in cancer care, which had started in 1791 when the brewer Samuel Whitbread endowed the first cancer ward in London for the care of moribund, inoperable cases. This started what was to be a long-lasting tradition of brewers supporting cancer care.

Apart from some minor benefit from the surgical removal of some tumours, 19th century treatments were seen as no better than 'wart charms'. This changed with the discovery of radioactivity in 1895. Almost immediately, the **Middlesex Hospital Radium Wing**, the fine red-brick façade in front of you that extends along much of Nassau Street, was built, partly funded by the Whitbread family. Further evidence of the ability of cancer care and research to attract benefactors can be seen above the entrance – Edward Myerstein, a wealthy novelist, provided a radiotherapy institute. Initially, supplies of radium, which emits radioactive radon gas, were very limited and expensive. Poor understanding of the dangers led to most of the staff who used the hospital's first X-ray machine dying from radiation-induced cancers. Facilities expanded along Nassau Street in 1910 thanks to a bequest from Henry Barnato. The façade, with a neo-classical portico, can be seen to the right of the Radium Wing. After World War I, supplies of radium improved when material was reclaimed from redundant gun-sights. This led to the establishment of additional radium institutes, one of which you will now visit.

Retrace your steps along Nassau Street, turn left and walk along Riding House Street. Just before crossing Great Titchfield Street you will pass, on your right, the **College of Naturopathic Medicine**, evidence of the enduring appeal of non-conventional therapies, which

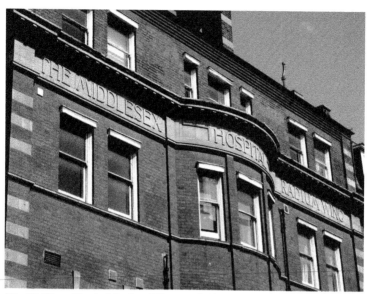

The Middlesex Hospital Radium Wing was built in 1900 to exploit the use of radioactivity (discovered only five years before) in the treatment of cancers. In 2012 only the façade survives, to be incorporated in a redevelopment of the site

have always been a feature of health care, despite the growth of scientific knowledge over the past century. The College has six branches in the UK that train people in a range of alternative therapies, all based on the notion of 'nature's own healing power'.

Continue to the end of Riding House Street. The last building on the right (Nos 1 and 3), just before All Souls Church, was built in 1914 and in 1928 became **Mount Vernon Hospital Radium Institute**. The hospital had been founded in 1859 in an elevated, rural location (in Hampstead). One of four specialist hospitals for tuberculosis (p. 218) established in London in the 19th century, it maintained an outpatient department in Fitzrovia (first in

Tottenham Court Road and later in Fitzroy Square) to be closer to those most likely to contract the disease. With London's outward spread, the hospital moved its inpatient facilities from Hampstead to Northwood in 1904. Then, with the decline in the incidence of TB, it shifted its focus to cancer in 1928. Repeated treatment with radiotherapy meant that an outpatient department in central London was convenient for patients so, for the next 22 years, the hospital maintained a radium institute here. However, by 1950 the hospital had diversified to serve the broader range of needs of its local population in north-west London. The continued existence of outpatient services in Fitzrovia had become an anachronism so it migrated out of London to join the main hospital.

Retrace your steps and turn left along Great Portland Street. After 50 m turn right into Langham Place. About 50 m on the left you will see a magnificent black and white tiled building that was the **Howard de Walden Nurses' Home**. It was built in 1900 as a residence and a club for private nurses who belonged to the Nurses' Cooperation, a company established by nurses in the 1890s to pursue fair remuneration for their work. The land and half the building cost was met by Lady Howard de Walden, from the family that owned (and continues to own) large swathes of Fitzrovia and Marylebone. Since the 1990s the building has housed a hotel and restaurant.

Return to Great Portland Street, cross over and walk about 400 m to the right and stop at the corner of Devonshire Street. Around here there were five hospitals that had contrasting destinies – two stayed in Fitzrovia by merging with a 'big beast' and two moved out of London. The fifth, the **London Throat Hospital**, was the last of five ENT hospitals (p. 82) to be established in the 19th century. It occupied a house (No. 206) on the opposite side of Great Portland Street from 1877 until 1913, when it merged with one of its rivals.

The corner where you are standing was occupied by the **National Dental Hospital**, an elegant custom-built three-storey building (demolished in the 1960s). The hospital and associated

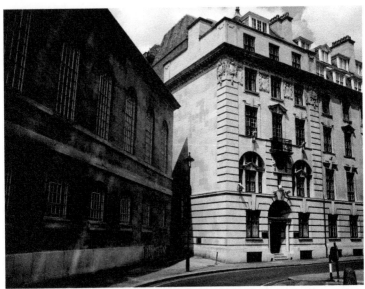

This 1914 building, behind John Nash's All Soul's Church, housed Mount Vernon Hospital's Radium Institute from 1928 to 1950

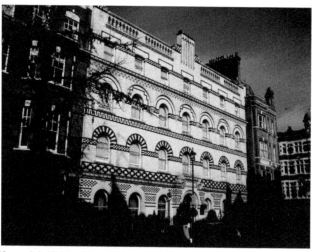

The Howard de Walden Nurses' Home (1900) was a residence and a club for private nurses who belonged to the Nurses' Cooperation, which sought fair remuneration for nurses. It is now a hotel

Metropolitan School of Dental Science had been established in 1859 in Cavendish Square. They moved to premises about 200 m south of here in 1861 and to this site in 1894. During the early 20th century, responsibility for the education of health care professions, including dentistry, was being taken on by the universities. In 1914 the National Dental College (as the school had been renamed) became part of the University of London, and the hospital merged with University College Hospital. This appeared to have secured its long-term future, a view that was strengthened when, in 1963, the hospital and college moved to new premises near University College Hospital in Mortimer Market. However, following a national

review of dentistry training and the hospital needs of Londoners, both were closed in the 1990s. The dental school merged with the Royal London Dental School at Whitechapel, and clinical services were transferred to the Eastman Dental Hospital.

Continue 50 m along Great Portland Street until you are outside the private Portland Hospital. The white stone building opposite, No. 234, was built in 1905 to accommodate the inpatients of the **Royal National Orthopaedic Hospital**. The hospital had started life in 1836 as the Spinal Hospital for the Cure of Deformities, initially only treating people in their own homes. Then, in 1856, it acquired the house directly behind the building you are looking at.

Walk 5

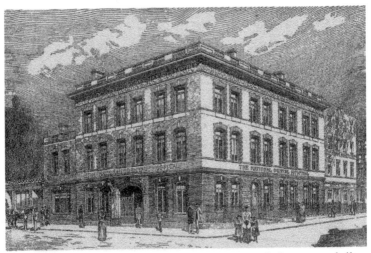

The elegant National Dental Hospital, built in 1894, was the first purpose-built dental hospital in England. It was demolished in the 1960s

At that time, it was competing with two other specialist hospitals – the Royal Orthopaedic and the City Orthopaedic Hospital. Attempts by the King's Fund (one of the hospitals' sources of income) to broker a merger were eventually successful, with the three merging on this site.

Many of the patients, particularly children, had TB. Pressure on space and the need for fresh air and sunshine led in 1922 to the opening of a country branch for chronic care and rehabilitation at Broccoli (now Brockley) Hill in Stanmore on the outskirts of London. In 1948 the hospital joined the NHS and the University of London located its postgraduate institute (p. 101) for orthopaedics here. By 1984 the building had become unsuitable for inpatient care, so its services were merged into the Middlesex

Hospital, while the Institute moved to Stanmore. The building now houses private consulting rooms for the Portland Hospital.

Continue along Great Portland Street and cross Euston Road. Turn left along the front of a small elegant terrace and then right through a gap in the centre of the terrace into Peto Place. Ahead of you on the left-hand side is a large, imposing three-storey polygonal building with stone-capped buttresses on the back of the nearby terrace. This was constructed in 1823 as a diorama (a precursor to the cinema). In 1930 the Red Cross Society took over the building and established a clinic for rheumatism, a condition that received little attention in the general hospitals. By 1936 it was seeing over 150,000 patients a year and had established a training school for masseurs and

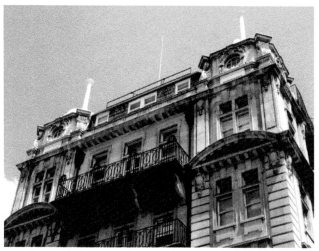

The upper floors of the Royal National Orthopaedic Hospital, built in 1905 to accommodate the merger of the three London orthopaedic hospitals

masseuses. In a throwback to the 19th century, nurses were trained in colonic irrigation in the belief that purging would remove toxins from the body. It was renamed the **Arthur Stanley Institute for Rheumatic Diseases** in 1948 after a senior society member who had been disabled after contracting rheumatic fever in his teens. When, in 1965, the Middlesex Hospital was looking to establish a rheumatology department, a merger suited both parties. The Institute moved to near the hospital, where it remained until its transfer to the new University College Hospital in 2005.

At the end of Peto Place is the Jerwood Medical Education Centre (part of the Royal College of Physicians). Leave via the covered exit to the right onto Albany Street. Cross over, walk past Melia White House and then cross Osnaburgh Street. Turn right and stop just before you reach Euston Road. The modern building beside you occupies the former site of **St Saviour's Cancer Hospital**, established in 1852. This was in a building set back from the road and included a chapel acquired from a Carthusian church in Bavaria. It was run by the Sisters of the Community of the Epiphany, Truro and was one of the first hospitals to specialise in caring for patients with cancer.

The absence of any clearly effective treatment for cancer at the time left the field open for all manner of therapies to be promoted. From 1873 the hospital was committed to a system of herbal medicine developed by an Italian count, Cesare Mattei, and known as electro-homeopathy. While influenced by Hahnemann, the founder of homeopathy, Mattei

Walk 5

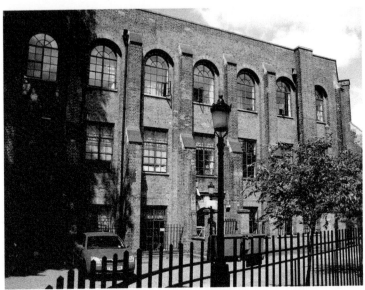

This 1823 diorama housed the Red Cross Institute for Rheumatic Diseases from its establishment in 1930 until its incorporation into and move to the Middlesex Hospital in 1965

believed that the fermented products of plants possessed additional energy, confusingly referred to as 'electro'. Its popularity can be gauged by the publication of 50 books on the subject between 1875 and 1930. Among the system's supporters was Mrs Booth, wife of the founder of the Salvation Army, who reported benefiting from pain relief when she was dying of cancer. In 1996 some enthusiasts reintroduced the system into the UK.

Like most voluntary specialist hospitals (p. 119), it struggled financially. By the 1890s the governors sought to widen its appeal by renaming it St Saviour's Hospital for Ladies of Limited Means. They were aiming at an emerging market, namely women who could pay a little but could not afford full nursing home charges. The contribution from patients became compulsory rather than optional. Despite such changes, the hospital gradually declined in size. In 1945, faced with rising costs and a fall in interest in electro-homeopathy, the hospital (together with the chapel) moved to Hythe in Sussex, where it has continued as a private general hospital.

Cross Euston Road, turn left and then second on the right into Conway Street, and stop as you enter Fitzroy Square. This architectural gem with many health care connections was laid out in 1790, although the north terrace (to your left) and the west terrace (on your right) were not constructed until the 1820s and

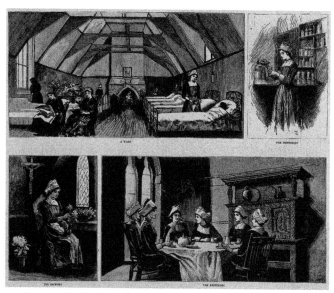

Scenes of nurses at St Saviour's Cancer Hospital in a ward, the dispensary, the sacristy and the refectory in 1886

Funding voluntary hospitals

Instigated in the early 18th century (apart from St Bartholomew's, St Thomas' and Bethlem with 16th century royal endowments), most voluntary funds came from *subscribers* who, in return for an annual donation, gained the right to determine who benefited (by issuing letters of recommendation to people). They were also eligible to be elected as governors of the hospital.

Donations and *endowments* were also sought. Most churches donated one Sunday collection each year and, in 1873, the Hospital Sunday Fund was established to 'rationalise' its distribution. Another productive source was concerts, balls and other 'charity' events. Large donations from rich philanthropists were usually for capital developments, sometimes extending to whole hospitals (e.g. the French Huguenot Hospital). Even larger amounts, as an endowment, could also meet the running costs (e.g. Guy's Hospital).

By the mid-19th century, working people were expected to contribute either by paying a small amount (a *co-payment*) – which would also discourage 'unnecessary' use – or in advance through *insurance schemes*, set up by Friendly Societies and churches. In addition, Hospital Saturday Funds based on collections in workplaces were set up. Although set up as donations, contributors expected to receive free treatment, and sometimes the organising committees (made up of working men) expected subscribers' rights in return for grants. Some dispensaries (p. 229) ran their own schemes (provident dispensaries), an approach later extended to hospitals with the development of Hospital Savings Associations.

Despite such initiatives, other sources of funds were still needed. In response, hospitals became more entrepreneurial: they established medical schools to attract student fees (although most went directly to the doctors); from the 1880s they established Nursing Institutions that hired out their trained nurses to private patients; they established lower cost convalescent homes (p. 92) to which long-term patients could be 'exported'; and they even exploited any street-level space by letting it for retailing. However, some ideas, such as charging people to visit patients outside normal visiting hours, were rejected.

By the 1890s many voluntary hospitals had no other option than to start accepting paying patients. This represented a fundamental change in policy that was opposed by some subscribers concerned that the working poor would suffer. 'Pay-beds' were only an option because there was a growing demand from two groups of people: those unable to afford home nursing and those living in lodgings or hotels. By 1893 about half the 63 voluntary hospitals in London had some pay-beds, although the building of entire private wings did not occur until the 1930s.

The other significant new source of finance was the King's Fund, based on an endowment created in 1897, which was soon contributing 10% of hospitals' income. The Fund felt this allowed it to influence hospital policy. Similarly, the Hospital Saturday Fund threatened to reduce its donation if a hospital did not introduce Lady Almoners (p. 85) to minimise 'abuse' by those not entitled.

Despite all these approaches, the 20th century saw increasing dependence on the state with financial support from local government. By mid-century, it was clear that survival was going to be dependent on central government funding, which arrived in the form of the NHS.

1830s, respectively. The other two terraces, designed by Robert Adam, were built in the 1790s.

Walk to your left along the north terrace and stop outside Nos 16 and 17. Aside from private madhouses, the first hospital in London successfully funded entirely by patient payments was established in these houses by the Home Hospitals Association in 1878. **Fitzroy House** was a nursing home with 24 beds that accepted both medical and surgical patients who were attended by their own private doctor. It aimed at those who were earning a living but did not have their own homes, such as governesses and those in lodgings for whom there was nowhere or no one to care for them when they were sick. In addition, the hospital provided somewhere for those living in the countryside to receive the attentions of the leading London doctors. In the 1930s it expanded to include No. 18, but it had to close in 1941 because of the war and never reopened.

Two houses further on (No. 14) is the only modern building in the square, the private Fitzroy Square Hospital. It was built in 1904 to accommodate **St Luke's Hospital for the Clergy**, a hospital established in Marylebone in 1892 to provide free care to Anglican clergy and their families. In addition to Anglican clergy, others who were allowed to use it included Church Army officers, members of monastic and conventual orders, overseas missionaries and licensed theological students. However, by 2006 it proved to be financially unsustainable, and the Church was forced to sell it in 2009 to a private hospital corporation.

Return to the corner of the square and walk along the west terrace to the south-west corner of the square. You pass No. 29, which from 1887 to 1898 was the home of George Bernard Shaw, whose sceptical views of the medical profession reflected the rather limited and dubious benefits of medicine at that time. The end house of the south terrace, No. 33, was the home of the **London Foot**

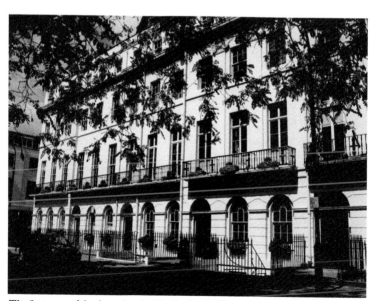

The first successful private hospital in England, Fitzroy House, was established at No. 16 in 1878 (on the far right), later expanded to the left into Nos 17 and 18, and eventually closed in 1941

Hospital from 1929 to 2004. It was established in 1912 in Soho and was unique in its focus on foot problems. It not only provided patient care, but also led the development of chiropody as a profession in the UK by establishing a medical society (p. 184), a journal and a training school. In 1948 it was incorporated into the NHS, and it expanded in 1959 when it acquired the house at the other end of this terrace, No. 40.

Walk along as far as No. 36, which from 1848 to 1859 was the initial headquarters of **St John's House**, the nursing sisterhood (p. 163) that, arguably, was the organisation that had the greatest influence on the development of health care in the 19th century. Starting with King's College Hospital in 1856, its staff and those of other sisterhoods transformed the state of voluntary general hospitals, making them clean, organised and safe havens for the sick.

Continue to the end of the terrace. Before being acquired by the London

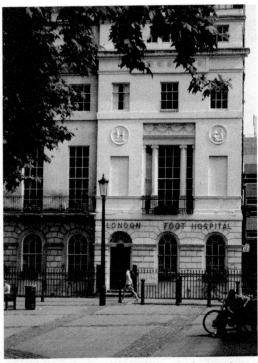

In 1929 the London Foot Hospital moved to this end-of-terrace house designed by Robert and James Adams in the 1790s and, despite the unsuitability of the building, stayed until 2004

Nursing sisterhoods

The middle of the 19th century witnessed a renewed emphasis in the Anglican Church to return to the Catholic tradition of undertaking nursing. Between 1840 and 1875, 42 sisterhoods were formed, each run by a Lady Superior who had some 'ladies of refinement' under her, the Sisters. In addition, there were probationers, working-class women who trained for a year to become nurses, and others who by virtue of their education were exempted from probation. Nurses worked among the poor, distributing spiritual, material and medical comforts, the forerunners of district nursing services. To fund this, the sisterhoods provided private nurses for the affluent, an arrangement that caused considerable tension given their religious motivation. However, exposure to wealthy homes showed them the advantages of hygienic conditions and fuelled their demand for higher standards of nursing.

Their nursing and organisational skills, together with a strong work ethic, became increasingly attractive to the governors of voluntary general hospitals (p. 148). In 1856 King's College Hospital went so far as to contract out its nursing services to St John's House Sisterhood, an arrangement that lasted for 11 years and was copied by other hospitals.

Despite inviting them in, the governors had three fears (all of which proved correct): that the sisters would proselytise; that their high expectations would lead to increased costs; and that their independence would challenge the authority of doctors and governors. From 1860 onwards, governors increasingly preferred the secular Nightingale schools because they could use their own probationer nurses as cheap labour and the schools were under the control of the hospital matron, and therefore the governors.

Walk 5

Foot Hospital, No. 40 had been the home of the London Skin Hospital from 1887, one of many skin hospitals (p. 132) in London. The demise of the Skin Hospital in 1959 gave the London Foot Hospital opportunity to expand. However, this was to prove only a short-term solution. Even though both No. 33 and No. 40 were modernised in 1980, improvements were limited by planning restrictions. The lack of lifts meant disabled patients had to be carried between floors. It was only a matter of time before the Foot Hospital would

go the way of its predecessor, the Skin Hospital. The only question was the inevitable one for small establishments – whether to merge locally with one of the big beasts or to migrate. The question was answered for them in 2003 when University College, of which the Foot Hospital School was a part, lost interest and the school was transferred to the University of East London. It was logical for the hospital to follow, which happened in 2004.

Before leaving the square, there is one more connection with health care to see. The penultimate house in the east terrace to your left (No. 2) was the home of another of the five ENT hospitals in central London, the **Metropolitan Ear, Nose & Throat Hospital**. It had been established by James Yearsley in 1838 near Piccadilly, devoted to ear and eye disease. This was a common combination at the time – Moorfields Eye Hospital started with a similar range of interests but chose to concentrate on eyes. Yearsley chose to concentrate on ears. The hospital occupied this house from 1911 but after World War II, faced with merging or moving, it chose the latter and acquired an old nursing home in Kensington. However, the move did not remove the pressure to merge, and in 1953 it was incorporated in St Mary Abbot's Hospital, Kensington. When that closed in 1985, it merged with Charing Cross Hospital in Fulham.

Leave the square by Grafton Way, and after about 100 m turn right into Whitfield Street. No. 108 on the left was the home of the first **family planning clinic** in the UK, established by the birth control pioneer Marie Stopes, one of the most influential people of the 20th century. Her advocacy of sex education helped liberate married couples (and women in particular) from ignorance and fear. The clinic had originally been set up in 1921 in Holloway but moved here after four years. Stopes advocated barrier methods (condoms and caps) and discouraged chemical

methods, famously saying, 'never put anything in your vagina that you would not put in your mouth'. While she was motivated by the desire to educate and empower people, she was unapologetic about also being a eugenicist. She believed birth control was needed to 'quell the stream of depraved, hopeless and wretched lives'. She even disinherited her son for marrying a woman 'handicapped' by glasses. As late as 1956, two years before her death, Stopes still held that a third of men should be sterilised, starting with the ugly and unfit.

Despite opposition from the Church and most of the medical profession, she survived threats of legal action. In 1930 local authorities were finally permitted to establish family planning services. Despite the rise of statutory services, private and charitable clinics continued. Since 1976 Marie Stopes International has been part of the largest non-NHS provider of family planning in the UK and is active in 43 other countries.

Continue along Whitfield Street, and after 200 m turn left into Howland Street. Cross over Tottenham Court Road, walk along to the end of Capper Street and stop. Here and in the surrounding streets are several buildings associated with the other 'big beast', University College Hospital. The first to look at is on the opposite side of Capper Street, the former **Royal Ear Hospital**, yet another of the ENT hospitals in central London.

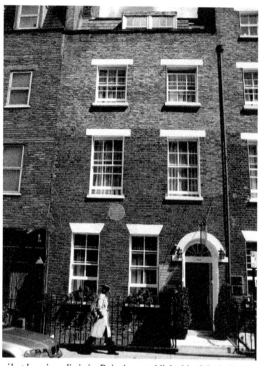

The first family planning clinic in Britain, established by Marie Stopes in Holloway, moved here after four years, in 1925

By the early 20th century, the voluntary general hospitals recognised the need for specialist departments. University College Hospital established an ENT department in 1905 and took the opportunity to enhance it by merging with the Royal Ear Hospital, based in Soho, in 1920. In 1926 the latter moved to the custom-built premises you can see today. As you can see from the plaque above the entrance, it was funded by Joseph Duveen (an art dealer). Initially, the wards had balconies on the western (right-hand) side, essential for recuperation from tuberculosis of the larynx, but later

these were enclosed to create space for more beds. In the basement there was a 'Silence Room' where acoustic experiments could be performed. Despite having such a splendid building, merger had started an inevitable journey to its disappearance as a distinct institution. It ended in 1997, when services were merged with the Royal National Throat, Nose and Ear Hospital in Gray's Inn Road. In 2012 the building was under threat of demolition.

Turn left into Huntley Street. The buildings lining both sides of the street were built for University College Hospital and, until recently, had been

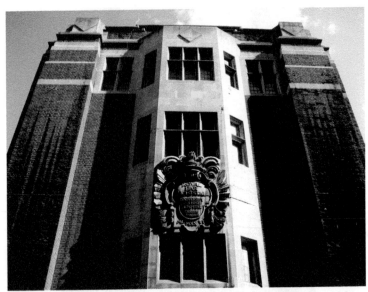

The fourth and final home of the Royal Ear Hospital, built in 1926 and paid for by Joseph Duveen, an art dealer. The hospital moved out in 1997, and in 2012 the building is threatened with demolition

constructed in the first half of the 20th century. In 2005 this started to change when, on the right side of the street, an institute for cancer research, designed by Jeremy Grimshaw, replaced a 1926 nurses' home and a nursing school. On the opposite side, a new cancer centre opened in 2012, replacing the 1926 **Obstetrical & Gynaecological Hospital**. The latter had been funded by the Rockefeller Foundation, demonstrating its ringing endorsement of University College Hospital as 'a medical educational centre of such standing and prestige as would secure the circulation of new ideas and methods throughout the British empire'. It was the first hospital in London to provide a 'flying squad' for emergency obstetric care in patients' homes. In 2001, it merged

with the Elizabeth Garrett Anderson Hospital (which had in turn already incorporated the Hospital for Women in 1989), creating the Elizabeth Garrett Anderson & Obstetric Hospital. You will see its new home in a moment.

As you continue along Huntley Street, the next building on the right (with an arched stone entrance with two columns and 'Nurses Home' carved in stone over the door) was the **Trained Nurses Institute**, built in 1907 as a home for University College Hospital-trained staff who were hired out to work privately in the community and generate income for the hospital. Having crossed University Street, turn round and look back. The modern red-brick building to the right of the new

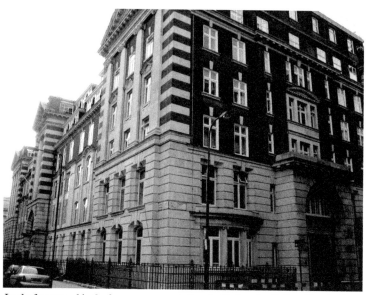

In the foreground is the former accommodation for University College Hospital's private nurses (when not hired out to patients' homes), and beyond is the Medical School, designed by Paul Waterhouse in 1907

cancer centre is yet another example of philanthropy: the **Rayne Institute** for medical research funded by Max Rayne, a property tycoon. Now look to the left along University Street and you can see how the Trained Nurses Institute forms a wing of a grand building that was designed by Paul Waterhouse in 1907 and paid for by Donald Currie, a shipping magnate. Most of the building housed the **Medical School**, although it also provided residential accommodation for medical and midwifery students training in the community.

Continue along Huntley Street.

On your left is the **Private Patients' Wing**, a very dull, lacklustre building that was constructed with funds

raised by the hospital's centenary appeal. It opened in 1937 and was connected to the main hospital building, on the other side of Huntley Street, by underground passages. Its most famous patient was George Orwell, who, in 1950, got married on his death bed here. The contrast with the dramatic and flamboyant red-brick building on the other side of the street could not be greater. This is the back of what was the main **University College Hospital** building from 1905 until 1995. Designed by Alfred Waterhouse (father of Paul), it replaced the original 1834 hospital building on this site. This was Waterhouse's last major commission; he died a year before its opening. Restricted by the small site, he met the contemporary requirements of plenty of natural light and fresh air (believed to be as helpful as the medical treatments administered) by adopting a cruciform design with the wards serviced from a central spine. It took eight years to build and can be considered the finest hospital building in London.

Standing in Huntley Street, you can see two of the four-storey ward blocks radiating out to each corner of the site, where there are towers topped with turrets. These 'sanitary towers' contained the patients' toilets and bathrooms, positioned there to minimise the risk of cross-infection. Note how the towers are separated from the wards by an open arcade, to reduce the risk of infection. Concern about adequate ventilation can also be seen in the perforated panels below each ward window. The cruciform structure stands upon a podium that contained outpatient clinics, diagnostic departments and other support services.

Walk on along Huntley Street and turn right into Grafton Way. After a few metres you can see on your right the old entrance for Skin, Eye & Dental Outpatients, and at the end of Grafton Street, on Gower Street, was the main Outpatients' Entrance. Look in through the glass doors to see the ornate marble and mosaic decorations that adorn much of the interior.

Cross Gower Street so that you can get a better view of the front of the building. Renaissance influences are evident: the arched windows in

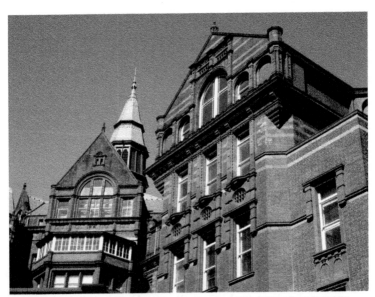

The most stunning hospital architecture in London, Alfred Waterhouse's 1905 cruciform building for University College Hospital

the top storey, classical mouldings to window surrounds, contrasting white bands (particularly on the entrance lodge) and the collection of chimneys, dormers and turrets at roof level. But the most striking feature today is the use of hard red-brick and terracotta, selected because of their resistance to erosion and looking as bright today as 100 years ago. The building was acquired by University College in 1995 and refurbished to recreate the original internal appearance and layout. It now houses a biomedical research institute and part of the medical school.

If you look to your right along Gower Street, you can see a 17-storey white and green building that forms the core of the new hospital, opened in 2005. In the foreground is the new home for the Elizabeth Garrett Anderson & Obstetric Hospital. It seems unlikely that this edifice will be being admired in 100 years.

As you walk along Gower Street towards the new hospital, note the building on your right (No. 136) on the corner with Gower Place. It was built in 1931 as **Lewis's Bookshop & Lending Library**, a service established in 1844 that specialised in medical books and which survived until the late 1980s. Note how Hippocrates gazes down on generations of medical students and doctors.

Stop at the end of Gower Street beside the entrance to Euston Square underground station. Looking across Euston Road you can see a green and white five-storey building. This used to be the Gower Hostel, providing accommodation for University College Hospital staff. The site to its left, where a modern, silvered office block now stands, was terraced houses in the 19th century. It was in the fourth house along in which the newly created University College established the **University Dispensary** in 1828 to provide clinical instruction for medical students, a function it provided until the North London Hospital (the original name of University College Hospital) opened in 1834 (on the site of Waterhouse's cruciform building).

Turn back to the underground station, which is embedded in the new **Wellcome Trust Headquarters**. This is not the first time this site has been connected with health care. From 1911 to 1935 the building next door to the station on Euston Road housed an example of people's faith in the therapeutic powers of water (p. 259). This was a **Sea-Water Dispensary**, established by a Parisian, Monsieur Quinton, who administered injections of diluted sea-water (or 'Plasma of Quinton' as he called it), claiming it had therapeutic and restorative powers. Following its demise, it was replaced by **St Margaret's Clinic for Tumours** (later the London Cancer Clinic), which migrated to Manchester for the duration of World War II. It is unclear what happened to it after its return to London in 1950.

Walk along Euston Road past the headquarters of the Wellcome Trust, a building that suggests the corporate headquarters of a multinational commercial company rather than a charity. The Trust is by far the largest non-commercial funder in the UK of medical research and research into the history of medicine. Beyond it is the imposing, granite and marble neo-classical **Wellcome Building**. It was built in 1932 for Henry Wellcome, who had made his fortune in the 1880s (with Silas Burroughs, a fellow American living in London) by manufacturing medicines in a new form that they called tabloids (tablets). This building was one of Wellcome's rewards, constructed to house the Wellcome Research Institution, a place of learning that he funded whose activities extended from laboratory research to archaeology and history, reflecting Wellcome's personal preoccupations. It was renamed The Wellcome Building in 1955 and houses the most extensive history of medicine library in Europe and exhibition space to promote public understanding of science and medicine.

Turn right down Gordon Street, alongside The Wellcome Building. The next building, now the University College London students' union, was originally a hotel, which, until the Friends House was built

in 1925 on the other side of the street, was on the corner of the extensive and attractive Euston Square. In 1919 the building was acquired by the Seamen's Hospital Society, a charity that had been established in 1821 'for the purpose of establishing a floating hospital for the assistance and relief of sick and helpless seamen'. Converted ships in the London docks were initially used, but in 1870 it came ashore, first at Greenwich and then also at Albert Dock. By 1919, when it decided to move to central London, it had expanded its brief to include tropical diseases and had established a specialist medical school. The **Hospital for Tropical Diseases** remained here until World War II forced it to return to a supposedly safer site in the East End. Meanwhile, the London School of Tropical Medicine had already moved to new premises a few hundred metres south in 1929. The hospital returned to central London in 1947 but, in 1998, like so many other specialist hospitals in the area, could not withstand the centrifugal force of University College Hospital.

The walk ends here, a short distance from Euston underground station.

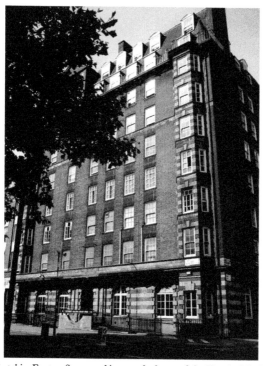

Built as a hotel in Euston Square, this was the home of the Hospital for Tropical Diseases, run by the Seamen's Hospital Society, from 1919 to 1940

Walk 6: From trades to professions

A key feature of the history of health care has been the battles between practitioners over the boundaries between each occupation: who they can treat, what treatments they can use, what they can charge for. Since 1750 each and every group has sought to distinguish itself from its competitors and to gain recognition as a 'profession'. Their objective has been to transform a service into an income-yielding property by gaining control of the market. Legal rights, self-regulation and formalised training were the tools that would give a group the social and economic security it sought. These developments, which have occupied practitioners over the past 200 years, have spawned numerous organisations, many of which have been located in this one small area of London, Marylebone. This walk traces the story of how the main health care professions – doctors, nurses, midwives, dentists – developed.

In 1750 there was only one group that enjoyed the benefits of professional status, the physicians. Few in number, they were educated at the exclusively Anglican universities of Oxford and Cambridge and had been granted a Royal Charter in 1518 to form a College. In contrast, the surgeons were still a City company, which had only recently (1745) separated from the barber-surgeons. And the apothecaries, who had separated from the grocers in 1617, were intent on distinguishing themselves from druggists and chemists, so as to emphasise their role as medical practitioners. Unlike physicians, training

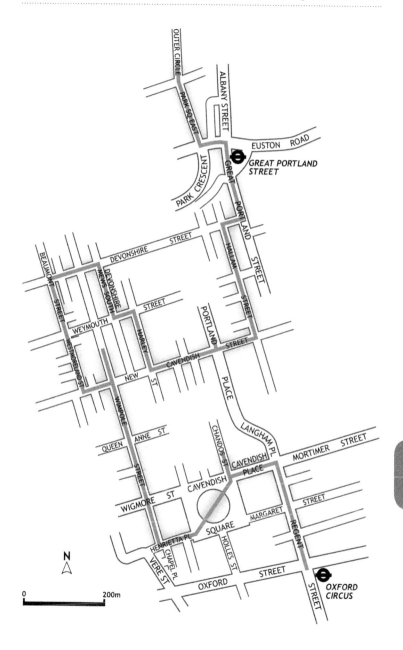

for surgeons and apothecaries was largely by apprenticeship, soon to be supplemented by attending a private anatomy school. The other trades had no formal preparation. The forerunners of dentists (tooth-pullers) learnt by experience, often from their parents, as did midwives. And nursing hardly registered as an occupation, consisting almost entirely of unskilled, menial tasks.

Until the 1720s the area north of Oxford Street was open country. Starting with Cavendish Square, the main thoroughfares of Harley Street, Wimpole Street and Portland Place were constructed, which linked London with the newly constructed east–west bypass, the New Road (Marylebone Road). For its first 100 years, this was a sought-after residential area. The affluent moved here from their homes in the City. However, by the middle of the 19th century, they started vacating Marylebone for the attractions of Belgravia and Kensington, and this provided the opportunity for the less prosperous to move in, in particular doctors.

Up until about 1840 the centre of the medical world in London was to the east in an area extending from Queen Square to Lincoln's Inn Fields, midway between their source of income, the homes of private paying patients in the West End, and the principal hospitals in the City (St Bartholomew's, St Thomas', Guy's, Bethlem). However, with changes to the social geography of London, it was vital that they did not get left behind. During the first half of the 19th century, new voluntary general hospitals (University College, Charing Cross,

King's College and the Royal Free) were established to the west of the City.

Doctors recognised the need to migrate west to stay near their sources of income. Marylebone became home not only to the leading practitioners, but also to the organisations that were to play key roles in the development of the health care professions. Hence, between about 1840 and 1920, the modern health care professions were defined and refined in this area. And to the present day this remains the political centre of the health care professions.

Granting a trade the status of a profession represents a deal between society (government) and an occupation. In return for gaining considerable freedom of self-determination and legal protection, the occupation pledges to act honestly and altruistically in the interests of the members of the public it serves and to advance both its subject and its personal knowledge and skills. Unlike other occupations, a profession controls who can join its privileged ranks by determining the entry requirements and minimum standards of practice; it receives legal protection that prevents non-members from practising; and it is allowed to regulate and police its members. To execute all these activities, each profession has needed to create five complementary organisations, each performing distinct functions:

- to establish and maintain professional standards – which are now largely the responsibility of royal colleges, although until 1930 only two existed: physicians (whose home you will see on this walk) and surgeons. Over the past 80 years, 11 more have been established, three of which are in Marylebone (nursing, midwifery and radiology).

- to guard their territories – for which professions established defence organisations, such as the Medical Protection Society, which was based in Marylebone. Their role was to prosecute unqualified intruders and to defend their members from unjustified or false accusations.

- to police their own members – for which regulatory bodies were established by Acts of Parliament: the General Medical Council in 1858; the Central Midwives Board in 1902; the General Nursing Council in 1919; and the Dental Board of the UK in 1921 – all four of which (and their successors) have been or still are located in Marylebone.

- to advance knowledge, which was led by professional societies. Some adopted a wide, general interest, such as the Medical Society of London and the Royal Society of Medicine (both in Marylebone), whereas others specialised (such as the X-ray Society). Apart from organising lectures and demonstrations, many published a journal, some of which survive to the present day.

And finally, just like other trades, professions are concerned with protecting and enhancing their members' financial well-being and employment rights. This initially depended on trades establishing their own benevolent associations to assist those members and their families who faced impoverishment through death or disablement. Examples include the Society for the Relief of Widows & Orphans of Medical Men (1788), the Benevolent Fund for Dentists (1883) and the Nation's Fund for Nurses (1917). With the establishment of trades unions, unlike the doctors who created a separate organisation (British Medical Association), the three other main professions chose to combine trades unionism with establishing and maintaining professional standards: the British Dental Association (since 1921), the Royal College of Nursing and the Royal College of Midwives.

Marylebone has been not only the centre of professional development in England, but also the location of two other significant developments in health care. One is the emergence of private hospitals. Until the mid-19th century, the affluent paid to be visited and cared for in their homes. This even extended to surgery, although the range of operations available at that time was very restricted. Three factors changed this. First, increasing numbers of people lived some distance from central London, too distant to be visited by expensive physicians and surgeons. So they required a 'home' in central London where they could stay while being treated. Also, social changes meant there were increasing numbers of single people in rented accommodation who had no family to care for them when they fell ill. Second, by the end of the 19th century, medical advances (most notably the availability of anaesthesia and aseptic practices) were permitting more complex treatments that required more than a kitchen table. And third, the well-justified fear of hospitals was diminishing as a result of the improvements pioneered principally by the nursing profession. All these factors contributed to the demand for hospitals and for paying patients.

Given the increasing concentration of medical men residing in Marylebone, it was inevitable that private facilities would develop here. Initially, doctors' homes doubled up as private consulting rooms for outpatients, while other houses were used as small private nursing homes. The massive growth in medical activity in Marylebone led to the area being referred to as Pill Island in the 1930s. The demand for more accommodation for clinical services, combined with the changing social aspirations of doctors, led them to move to live in the suburbs and home counties. Entire houses could now be given over to consulting rooms, enabling even more doctors to work here. Meanwhile, the small nursing homes gave way to private hospitals, some having as many as 200 beds and state-of-the-art high-tech equipment, such as the Harley Street Clinic and the Portland Hospital (both of which you will see).

Marylebone also illustrates the important role that charity has played in supporting health care research (Novartis Foundation) and policy and service development (Nuffield Trust and King's Fund). Like the other organisations already mentioned, they too needed to be near the centre of the health care world, here in Marylebone.

The walk starts at Oxford Circus underground station. Leave the station by Exit 4 to the north side of Oxford Street and west side of Regent Street. Walk north along Regent Street as far as the second set of traffic lights, Cavendish Place. Cross Cavendish Place and turn left. Take the first on the right, Chandos Street, and stop after about 30 m, opposite the home of the **Medical Society of London**.

Throughout Europe in the late 18th century, the medical profession (p. 200) started founding medical societies (p. 184), organisations that brought people together to facilitate and encourage scientific, professional and social communication. The Medical Society of London was the first general society in England (rather than one focused on a particular hospital or specialty). It was founded in 1773 by, among others, John Coakley Lettsom, a Quaker physician and philanthropist who also helped establish the first voluntary dispensaries (p. 229) and the Royal Sea Bathing Hospital at Margate. One of the founding aims was to bring the three warring factions – physicians, surgeons and apothecaries – together. Initially based in the City, the Society moved west in 1850 and to this location in 1871. It originally occupied only the right-hand house, No. 11, then acquired No. 12 and then extended into the back gardens in 1892. The result is the long, low, stuccoed building with Corinthian pilasters. Despite both the defection of a disaffected group of members who left to form an alternative society

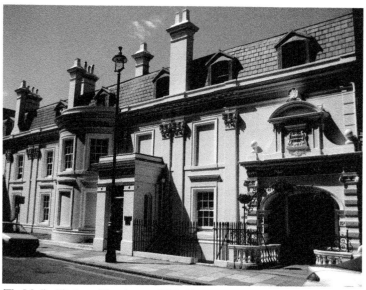

The Medical Society of London, established in 1773, created its current home in Chandos Street in the 1880s by modifying two Georgian houses

(more on that in a moment) and the establishment of many other organisations, remarkably this society has survived, although today it has only about 500 members.

Over the years, the Society has assisted other charitable medical organisations. One has been the **Society for the Relief of Widows & Orphans of Medical Men**, founded in 1788 by a small group of doctors (including Lettsom) who perceived the need for a benevolent fund for the widows and orphans of colleagues who had fallen on hard times. However, they struggled to get members, given the requirement that they make quite substantial donations. They initially met in a coffee house, but from 1893 to 1971 they were taken in by the Medical Society of London. Despite membership never being more than about 300, they were able to help about 50 widows and a few orphans each year. Although membership declined after World War II, it continues to function, once again finding sanctuary here in this building.

Before leaving, note the magnificent Chandos House at the far end of the street. Designed by Robert and James Adam in 1770, for much of the last 40 years it has provided additional space for overnight accommodation and meetings for the other long-established medical society, the Royal Society of Medicine (the RSM, which you will visit in a short while).

Walk 6

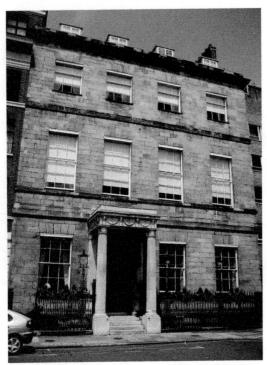

One of the Adam brothers' finest townhouses, Chandos House, has provided additional accommodation for the Royal Society of Medicine since 1964

Return to Cavendish Place, turn right and almost immediately cross over onto the broad pavement in Cavendish Square. Stop and turn round to look at the north side of the square, dominated by two elegant Palladian-style stone-fronted houses in the centre, built in 1770. The road between them was to preserve an urban axis running from Hanover Square (south of Oxford Street). In practice, a mews and a convent were built behind the houses, closing off the intended axis. The convent became the home of the **King's Fund** in 1993.

The King's Fund was established in 1897 by the future Edward VII (encouraged by Henry Burdett, the leading hospital reformer of the period) to help with funding voluntary hospitals (p. 159) in London. He pledged to match any other donations to establish an endowment, the interest from which could be given each year to hospitals. The pace and scale of the fund-raising was remarkable, reflecting the social advantages of being seen by the royal family to have contributed. Within a decade the Fund stood at £227,000, and interest from it was providing 10% of the income of London's voluntary hospitals.

The trustees realised the potential influence this gave them, and this heralded the first attempt at the strategic planning of voluntary hospitals in London. It paralleled the work of the Metropolitan Asylums Board (p. 179), which, since 1867, had been coordinating the development of public hospitals for infectious diseases, mental illness and mental subnormality. To inform their decisions, King's Fund trustees began inspecting and assessing the performance of hospitals. Their attempts at facilitating the amalgamation of voluntary specialist hospitals (p. 119) met both with success (orthopaedics) and failure (ENT hospitals), as did encouraging some voluntary general hospitals (p. 148) to move away from central London. Since the start of the NHS, the Fund has supported innovations in the organisation of services,

the training of managers and contributed to policy debates. While independent of government, its patron remains a senior member of the royal family who takes an active interest in the Fund's affairs.

Turn now to one of the buildings on the east side of the square, No. 5. In the 1850s people from a variety of backgrounds offered to pull teeth. The need for some form of regulation and registration accompanied by formal training was increasingly recognised by leading practitioners, although they were divided into two distinct groups as regards how to proceed: the 'Memorialists' and the 'Independents' (mirroring a similar division in France). In 1856 the former established the Odontological Society, an organisation that worked closely with the Royal College of Surgeons to lobby parliament to have dentistry (p. 187) covered by the proposed Medical Act.

Metropolitan Asylums Board

By the 1850s criticism of the inadequacies of the Poor Law system to meet the needs of the poor was mounting. The National Association for the Promotion of Social Science, set up by critics such as Louisa Twining, reported on the conditions in the workhouse infirmaries (p. 54) and established the Workhouse Visiting Society in 1858 to campaign for improvements. Over the following decade, many joined in the call for reform, including Charles Dickens, Florence Nightingale and The Lancet. In

1866 the Association for Improvement of the Infirmaries of London Workhouses was formed, which called for the establishment of six 1,000-bed hospitals with properly trained staff, funded centrally.

The Metropolitan Poor Act passed a year later allowed radical reforms to go ahead. Existing Poor Law Unions and parishes were to amalgamate into six Sick Asylum Districts, each one required to build a hospital funded from a London-wide fund that would redistribute money from affluent to poorer areas of the city. The need to separate the sick, insane, incurable and children was accepted. And the whole enterprise was to be centrally managed by the Metropolitan Asylums Board (MAB). In addition, infectious disease hospitals (p. 78) were to be provided, as were asylums for 'imbeciles' (those who were educationally subnormal).

In practice, the cost of six large new general hospitals proved too much, and after two were constructed (Central London District and Poplar & Stepney District) the programme ceased and the Unions making up the other districts were allowed to redeploy existing buildings. Within ten years, five fever and smallpox hospitals were established on the edge of the city. To support the hospitals, an ambulance (p. 106) system was established with six stations positioned strategically around the city. For the first time, a coordinated, state-run hospital system existed.

Similar central planning led, in 1870, to the creation of two large asylums for 'imbeciles' (Leavesden and Caterham) and a separate facility for children (initially in Hampstead, and then at Darenth near Dartford). Further hospitals, schools and 'training colonies' followed over the next few decades.

Up until 1890 the provision of hospitals in London remained on two separate tracks – workhouse infirmaries for paupers and voluntary hospitals for the working poor. In 1891 this changed when an Act permitted the admission of non-paupers to the MAB fever and smallpox hospitals. Significantly, the cost of care for all patients was to be met from the public purse. One consequence was the need for expansion, and five additional hospitals were built.

In the early years of the 20th century, the MAB had to meet two additional challenges. First, the growing importance of TB (p. 218) led to the Board establishing sanatoria for 'open air' treatment. Mostly, existing buildings were acquired and converted. Second, recognition of the importance of venereal disease (p. 123) led to the MAB establishing two hospitals – the Institution for Venereal Diseases for women and St Margaret's Hospital in Kentish Town for infants with ophthalmia neonatorum acquired from their infected mothers.

By the time the MAB handed over its responsibilities to the London County Council in 1930, the long-term basis for a modern health system had been established.

Meanwhile, the Independents formed the Society of Dentists and set up a training body, the College of Dentists, as a rival to the Royal College of Surgeons. They were opposed to the Memorialists' readiness to be subsumed within surgery, preferring to retain dentistry's independence from doctors. In 1859 the Independents established the **Metropolitan School of Dental Science** here at their headquarters at 5 Cavendish Square, and in 1861 they established the National Dental Hospital in Great Portland Street. However, they recognised that the Memorialists had the upper hand because, as part of the Royal College of Surgeons, they had exclusive rights to license dentists. Few potential dentists were going to be attracted to study with the Society if it did not result in obtaining a licence to practise. A truce was essential. Amalgamation of the societies took place in 1863, the same year that the Metropolitan School moved from here to the National Dental Hospital. While this appeared to settle the issue once and for all, in the 21st century some dentists are once again questioning the wisdom of the profession remaining as a faculty of the Royal College of Surgeons rather than seeking independence with its own royal college.

Enter the gardens in the middle of the square and cross diagonally and exit. Opposite is No. 20, the **Royal College of Nursing** (RCN). As happened with dentistry, the quest for improved status and conditions led to two factions in nursing: a more radical one seeking independence and self-determination, and a more cautious one accepting less autonomy. The former view was first manifest by the establishment of the British Nursing

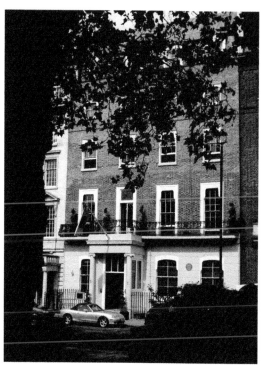

The Society of Dentists, formed in 1856, established the Metropolitan School of Dental Science in this house in Cavendish Square in 1859

Walk 6

Council in 1887 (which became the Royal British Nursing Association in 1899). Led by the formidable Ethel Bedford Fenwick, it formed a register to which only nurses of at least three years' experience were admitted. It advocated the development of nursing as a profession independent of medicine. As such, it distinguished between specialised nursing skills requiring training and unskilled domestic duties.

In contrast, the College of Nursing, established in 1916, was more inclusive, recognising and accepting the full range of duties performed by nurses. Its aims were to promote better training, encourage uniformity across the 1,500 nursing schools in England, and maintain a register of proficient nurses. With the help of their greatest benefactor, Lady Cowdray, they established a benevolent fund (the Nation's Fund for Nurses) to provide for nurses whose health had been damaged by World War I. She also purchased 20 Cavendish Square (the penultimate house on this side of the square at the time) from Herbert Asquith (the Prime Minister), to serve as a headquarters for the College and as a residential club for nurses and other professional women.

The tension between the two factions reached a head during the debates around the 1919 Nurses Act. Government was wary of relinquishing too much independence to nurses but, along

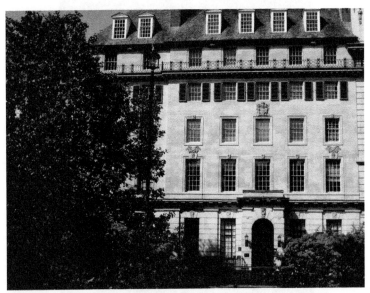

The College of Nursing initially occupied the penultimate house in the 18th century terrace on the west side of Cavendish Square but, having acquired adjacent properties, united them in the 1930s within the building you see today

with hospital managers, was concerned to stem the growth of trades unionism, a threat that would increase if all aspirations of professional status were denied. The College of Nursing seemed to offer the least worst option. The Act created a General Nursing Council (whose headquarters you will visit later) composed of nine lay people, ten members of the College and only four from Bedford Fenwick's Association. Nursing was the last of the main health care professions to gain legal status, some eight years after parliament had granted protection for domestic animals.

The expanded role for the College led to the need for more space. In 1928–30 the house on the corner, No. 21, and two properties behind it in Henrietta Place were bought. The current building was created in the 1930s by retaining the finest internal features of the two 18th century houses in the square, building behind them and enveloping the ensemble in the façade you see today. In 1939 the college received a Royal Charter. However, unlike the medical royal colleges (p. 194), which concentrate on professional standards and education, the RCN combined these with a trade union role. This culminated in their consideration of the use of industrial action on occasions during the last few decades. Meanwhile, the late-19th century debate between inclusivity and exclusivity continues into the 21st century within the RCN.

Cross over to John Lewis department store and walk to the right along Henrietta Place. Note the nursing motifs, such as bandaging and a lamp, on the side of the RCN building. The next building is the home of the **Royal Society of Medicine**. In 1805 a group of members of the Medical Society of London objected to the high-handed behaviour of the president, Dr James Sims, who after 19 years in post showed no sign of giving up office. So they broke away and formed the Medical & Chirurgical Society of London. Among them was Dr Peter Mark Roget, later to find fame by devising the thesaurus that bears his name. Similar to the society they had left, their aim was to provide a venue 'for the purpose of conversation on professional subjects, for the reception of communications and the formation of a library'. They occupied several premises in and around Holborn (the centre of medical London at that time), before moving west to Berners Street (near the Middlesex Hospital) and then Hanover Square. They also acquired the 'Royal' prefix, which must have annoyed the longer established Medical Society of London. By 1900 their long-term future as the premier medical society was secured as a result of their incorporation of 16 specialist societies, and they needed larger premises. This custom-built home opened in 1910.

Although its official address has always been 1 Wimpole Street, you can see that its original main entrance was in Henrietta Place

Medical societies

In the mid-18th century, there were few opportunities for practitioners to learn from one another's experiences and ideas. In Italy the Accademia dei Lincei had been established in 1603, and the Royal Academy of Surgery was founded in Paris in 1731. In Britain, scientists had established the Royal Society in 1653.

The first medical society in London, Guy's Hospital Physical Society, was established in 1771. Like many of the earliest societies, it was founded by a group of students in a voluntary general hospital, with the support of hospital governors and honorary medical staff. Many more followed, some focused on a particular hospital, others on a specialty, religion, employment or geographical area. Of the 30 established by 1850, the Medical Society of London (1773) and its breakaway, the Medical & Chirurgical

Society (1805), were to prove the most influential. Doctors were not alone in forming societies: the Pharmaceutical Society and the Matron's Aid Society were just two examples formed by other professions.

The aim of societies was met through holding meetings, establishing libraries and founding journals that reported the societies' proceedings. Financed by members' subscriptions, the largest acquired their own premises and offered the facilities of a gentleman's club. For doctors not associated with a hospital, societies provided their only contact with colleagues.

Some societies have survived, others were transformed into royal colleges, but many ceased after several decades as undergraduate schools and other providers of education and exchange emerged.

(with only a side door in Wimpole Street). However, the members craved the social cache of a Wimpole Street address. The building has a small albeit monumental façade with four recessed giant Doric columns and a fanciful entrance, above which it was intended to place a large sculpture. An extra storey was added in 1952.

Cross over to the Royal Society of Medicine and turn down Wimpole Street. You can see how the RSM expanded in the 1980s by incorporating part of the neighbouring postal sorting office, and created a new main entrance.

The RSM continues to pursue the aims of the founders by holding hundreds of meetings each year, publishing books and journals, and providing a London 'home' for members from afar.

Walk along Wimpole Street, crossing Wigmore Street and Queen Anne Street. Built in the 1720s it contains numerous connections with health care, some of which are commemorated with plaques. Continue as far as No. 63–64 on the left, the home of the **British Dental Association**, a rather undistinguished building compared with its Georgian neighbour.

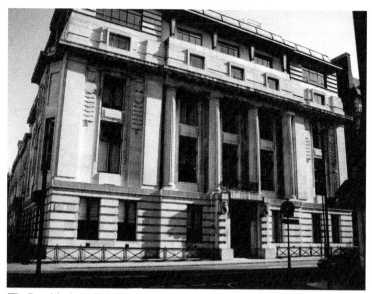

The Royal Society of Medicine's custom-built home (1910), with its original monumental main entrance in Henrietta Place (despite claiming a Wimpole Street address)

Despite the Royal College of Surgeons having been granted control over dental qualifications in 1858, a plethora of tradesmen still practised tooth-pulling, threatening dentists' aspirations to attain professional status. Doctors were generally unsupportive, with the *British Medical Journal* expressing the view that 'Medicine is a profession. Dentistry is largely a business'. Also, they could expect no help from the royal colleges in Scotland and Ireland, which exploited the situation by the unrestricted sale of licences to 'druggist's assistants, hairdressers, tobacconists and barbers', a useful source of income. However, lobbying led to the Dentists' Act of 1878, which established the British Dental Association (BDA) with all five

roles of controlling entry to the profession (maintaining a register), defending the profession from intruders (prosecuting unregistered practitioners), defending members' interests, supporting members 'who have fallen on evil times' (by means of a benevolent fund) and protecting the public (policing the members). As you will see in a minute, the BDA was relieved of some of these responsibilities in 1921, leaving it to concentrate on looking after the interests of its members, a role similar to that of the British Medical Association. The BDA moved home four times before, in 1966, buying two derelict Georgian houses here, demolishing them and building the replacement you see today. It houses a dental museum that is open to the

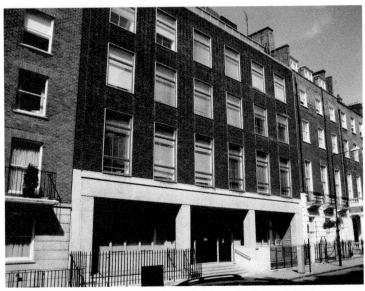

In 1966 the British Dental Association replaced two derelict Georgian houses (similar to those beyond it) with this drab, lifeless building

public (www.bda-dentistry.org.uk/museum).

Continue along Wimpole Street as far as No. 37 on the right, the home of the **General Dental Council**, and an example of the woeful planning controls in place in the late 1950s. In 1921 parliament was concerned that the interests of patients might be compromised if they were to be protected by the same body as that responsible for protecting the interests of dentists, the BDA. So a separate body, the Dental Board of the UK, was created to police the profession, which, as you have just seen, left the BDA to protect the professions' interests. Much to the chagrin of many dentists, the Board was in effect a subcommittee of the doctors' regulator, the General Medical Council. It was not until 1956 that the dentists gained independence when the General Dental Council was formed, which has occupied this building since 1960. As of 2012, unlike the doctors, nurses and allied health professions who each have their own regulatory bodies, the General Dental Council regulates all dental professions – dentists, hygienists, nurses and therapists. Like the other regulators, professionals make up only half the membership of the Council.

Retrace your steps along Wimpole Street and turn right into New Cavendish Street. Turn right along Westmoreland Street and walk about 70 m where you will see, on the right, the **National Heart Hospital**. It is one of the few hospitals to have moved from the NHS to the private

Dentistry

Until the mid-19th century, people from a variety of backgrounds offered to pull teeth. There was no delineation between trained dentists and others. While the need for some form of regulation and registration accompanied by recognised training was acknowledged by all the leading practitioners, they were split over the way forward between the Memorialists and the Independents (mirroring a similar division in France).

The Memorialists established the Odontological Society in 1856 and worked closely with the Royal College of Surgeons to lobby parliament to have dentistry covered by the proposed Medical Act. In 1859 they established the Dental Hospital of London (later the Royal Dental Hospital), along with the London School of Dental Surgery as a place for training (initially in Soho Square and later in Leicester Square).

Meanwhile, the Independents formed the Society of Dentists and set up a training body, the College of Dentists, as a rival to the Royal College of Surgeons. They were opposed to the Memorialists' readiness to be subsumed within surgery, instead wanting to retain dentistry's independence from doctors. In 1859 they established the Metropolitan School of Dental Science at their headquarters in Cavendish Square, and in 1861 the National Dental Hospital was established in Great Portland Street.

Inevitably, the Independents accepted defeat because the Memorialists, as part of the Royal College of Surgeons, had exclusive rights to license dentists. Few potential dentists were going to be attracted to study somewhere that did not result in obtaining a licence to practise. A truce was essential and was achieved in 1863.

By the 1870s there was a call for the formation of a national dental association and the establishment of dentistry as a profession. This ambition was not shared by everyone. The *British Medical Journal* took the view that 'Medicine is a profession. Dentistry is largely a business'. Despite this, lobbying culminated in the Dentists Act of 1878, which required dentists to be licensed and on the Dentists Register, run by the newly established British Dental Association (BDA).

Much of the early work of the BDA involved prosecuting illegal practitioners. Despite this, unregistered practitioners continued to outnumber the registered, and there was not even any guarantee that those registered were *bona fide*. In 1882 the BDA claimed that the Scottish and Irish royal colleges made money by selling licences to 'druggist's assistants, hairdressers, tobacconists, and barbers'. Whether true or not, such stories encouraged scepticism among doctors, who still questioned whether dentistry was truly a profession.

Public pressure finally led to more stringent control under the 1921 Dentists Act, which restricted practice to registered persons and created the Dental Board of the UK to administer the register. The latter was in effect a subcommittee of the General Medical Council. This freed the BDA from policing the profession and allowed it to become the dentists' trade union.

Walk 6

sector and back again, reflecting the changing fortunes of the two sectors. It was established in 1857 as the Hospital for Diseases of the Heart, a small voluntary specialist hospital, the first in the world dedicated to cardiovascular disease. It had three homes before moving to purpose-built premises here in 1914 as the National Heart Hospital. In 1948 it was incorporated into the NHS, and the University of

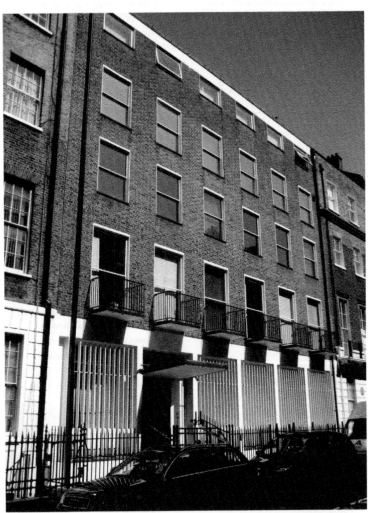

The General Dental Council gained independence from the General Medical Council in 1956, and has since 1960 occupied this building with its unsightly, barred ground-floor windows

London located its postgraduate institute (p. 101), the Institute of Cardiology, here. The first heart transplantation in the UK took place here in 1968. Despite this, its small size and isolation led to its services being moved to the Brompton Hospital, Kensington, in 1991, and the hospital was closed. It reopened as a private hospital in 1994 after a complete rebuild that preserved only the façade. But it struggled financially due, according to supporters, to a conflict of interests in which a leading private insurer (PPP) refused to recognise it and forced its insurees to be treated in other hospitals, which it just happened to own. In an unprecedented move, the hospital was bought back by the NHS in 2001 to become the cardiac department of University College Hospital.

Continue along Westmoreland Street, cross Weymouth Street and into Beaumont Street. Stop opposite Clarke's Mews on the right. The grand red-brick and stone six-storey building on the other side of the road was, from 1945 to 1967, the home of **The Tavistock Clinic**. Founded in 1920 in Tavistock Square, this provided mental health treatment based on psychological approaches. This was at a time when psychologists were seeking recognition to practise alongside medically qualified psychiatrists. It moved here to a shabby, derelict building that had been a private nursing home. A measure of its

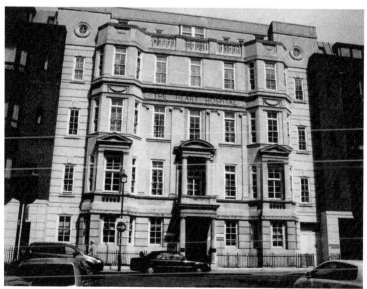

The National Heart Hospital, established in 1857 as the first hospital in the world dedicated to cardiovascular disease, occupied these purpose-built premises from 1914 to 1991.

success was that the Clinic was incorporated into the NHS in 1948. Alongside, it created a charitable company (the Tavistock Institute of Human Relations) to manage its research, consultancy and training activities. By 1967, when the Clinic moved to purpose-built premises in Swiss Cottage, it was well respected, and clinical psychologists were well established as an essential health care profession.

After the Tavistock Clinic left, the building was taken over by its neighbour, the **King Edward VII Hospital**, which occupies the rest of that side of the street. Walk along until you are opposite the entrance to the hospital. It was established in 1899 by two Jewish sisters, Agnes and Fanny Keyser, motivated by the plight of sick and wounded officers returning from the Boer War. They initially turned their home in Belgravia into a hospital and raised funds from 24 friends who agreed to make annual donations. In 1904 they acquired separate premises and gained the support of Edward VII as patron. Access was restricted to officers in the armed services who had served for at least five years and their spouses, widows and widowers.

In 1948 the hospital moved to purpose-built premises here. Funding continued to rely on donations from 'friends', now numbering several thousand, although patients were also expected to contribute. Access was widened to include all ex-service personnel, irrespective of rank, and even civilians were accepted if they were

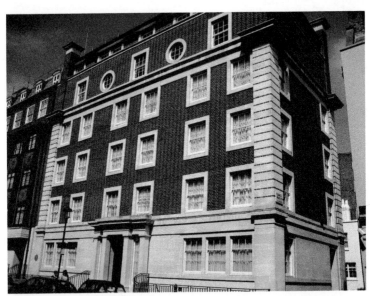

The Tavistock Clinic moved here in 1945, from converted stables in Bloomsbury, to occupy this ex-nursing home in Beaumont Street until 1967

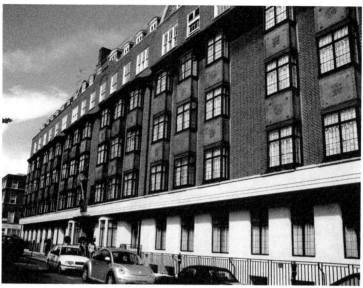

The King Edward VII Hospital, established in Belgravia in 1899 for wounded army officers returning from the Boer War, has occupied these purpose-built premises since 1948

prepared to pay – a situation that pertains today.

Walk on and when you reach Devonshire Street, stop and look at the four-storey red-brick building on the other side of the road (No. 23, Elizabeth House). From 1947 to 1951 it provided temporary accommodation after World War II for the **Hospital for Tropical Diseases**. Since then it has provided residential accommodation for staff from University College Hospital, and since 1991 it has also housed a crèche for the children of hospital staff.

Turn right along Devonshire Street, and after about 100 m turn right into Devonshire Mews South and then first left into Weymouth Street. On the other side of Weymouth Street, you will see one of

several private hospitals in the area, **The Harley Street Clinic**. Despite its name, its main entrance is actually in Weymouth Street. It is not the only institution to use the street name flexibly – Harley Street house numbers extend 50 m and three doors down some of the side streets!

Cross Harley Street and stop outside No. 90 on the opposite side. This 1910 building stands on an important site in the history of health services. From the 1840s onwards, small nursing homes were established throughout Marylebone, often by senior, experienced nurses from the major voluntary hospitals. One such was the **Establishment for Invalid Gentlewomen during Temporary Illness**, founded in 1850 in the house that stood on

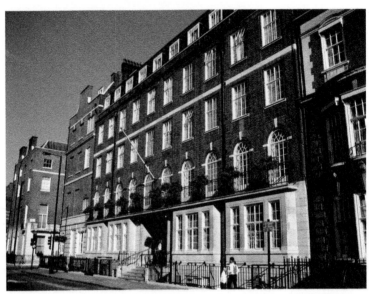

One of several private hospitals in Marylebone, the main entrance to the Harley Street Clinic is actually in Weymouth Street

this site. What marked this nursing home out from all others was the appointment, in 1853, of a 33-year-old nurse, Florence Nightingale, as Lady Superintendent. This was her first appointment. Despite occupying the post for only just over a year, she instituted several reforms. First, she threatened to resign if Catholic and Jewish patients were barred from being admitted. Then she had hot water piped to every floor, had a lift installed to bring patients' food to the floors and had bells installed so patients could summon nurses. She also instituted quarterly reports to the governors that covered improvements to the facilities, the cost of delivering services and the numbers of admissions and discharges. She was one of the first, if not the first, person to consider

monitoring the outcome of care in a systematic way.

Her interest in and promotion of statistical monitoring was to be one of several lasting and profound contributions to the development of health care, an activity that started in this small institution. She also found time to supervise the nursing of cholera victims at the Middlesex Hospital. After Nightingale's departure to Scutari to nurse soldiers from the Crimean War, the Establishment for Invalid Gentlewomen continued, employing such splendidly named staff as the Honourable WC Spring Rice as treasurer and Miss Tidy as Lady Superintendent. In 1910 it moved to Paddington and was later renamed the Florence Nightingale Hospital for Gentlewomen, eventually becoming

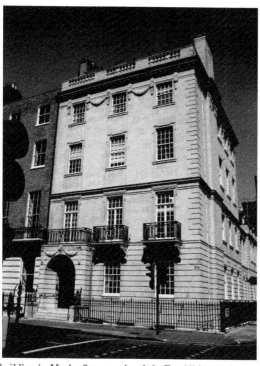

This 1910 building in Harley Street replaced the Establishment for Invalid Gentlewomen During Temporary Illness that, in 1853, provided Florence Nightingale with her first opportunity to improve hospitals

a private hospital specialising in acute psychiatric care.

Cross Weymouth Street and walk along Harley Street as far as No. 84. Some of the original early-18th century houses remain (such as the brick façades on the other side of the street), but repeated and extensive rebuilding has resulted in a mix of styles. In the 19th century, Benjamin Disraeli described the street as 'flat, spiritless and dull'. The same could not be said of the activities of some early medical residents. If you had stood here in the 1830s, you would have seen ladies' carriages blocking the street. They were flocking to see

John St John Long (known as the King of the Quacks, despite being a registered doctor), who ran a practice for wealthy women patients here at No. 84. Inside, he would ask patients to inhale from yards of mysterious pink tubing filled with a potent gas. This apparently decreased their resistance to his 'laying on of hands'. Following the death of two patients, he was convicted of manslaughter but fined only £250. Fortunately for other unsuspecting patients, he died prematurely at 36 from tuberculosis.

Despite such notorious cases, Harley Street proved an irresistible location for the leading doctors of

Walk 6

the mid-19th century. There was easy access to most of the new voluntary general hospitals where they held honorary appointments, and it was convenient for patients arriving from out of London at the great new railway termini. The growth in consulting rooms was phenomenal. From a dozen doctors in the 1860s, the number grew to 157 in 1900. The limited number of available houses led to multiple lettings from the 1920s, so that by 1985 there were over 800 and by 2003 over 1,400 doctors with rooms here. Position in the street was also important. In 1886 Sir John Tweedie was warned by colleagues that he would be committing professional suicide by moving too far from Cavendish Square.

Continue along Harley Street, turn left into New Cavendish Street and stop outside No. 59, the home of **The Nuffield Trust**. Established in 1940 with an endowment from William Morris (Viscount Nuffield), The Nuffield Provincial Hospitals Trust was a charity aimed at coordinating the development of health services outside London. (London had benefited from attempts at coordination by the Metropolitan Asylums Board since

1867 and the King's Fund since 1897.) Initially based in Oxford, it moved to Regent's Park in 1960 and here in 1993. The Trust's emphasis has always been to promote improvements in the organisation of services. Being financially independent of government, it fulfils an important role in terms of strategic thinking and independent commentary on health care in the UK.

There are three other buildings in the vicinity that have also been associated with health care. First, No. 61 next door was the home of the 19th century architect Alfred Waterhouse, responsible for arguably the finest hospital building in London, the 1905 University College Hospital. Second, No. 63 was the headquarters of the **British Psychoanalytical Society** from the 1940s until 1999. Founded in 1913 by Ernest Jones, its aim, like that of most medical societies, was to establish and safeguard professional standards. A journal was established, and the Institute of Psychoanalysis was set up in 1924 to provide training, development of theory and practice, publications, lectures and a library.

And the third is the large house with a blue front door on

Royal colleges

In 1511 the small number of Oxbridge-educated physicians obtained exclusive rights to practise medicine. Inspired by his observations in Italy, Thomas Linacre led the establishment of a College of Physicians in 1518. His aim was a royal and academic body that would control entry to the profession

and would, incidentally, be exclusively Protestant, given that Catholics were excluded from Oxbridge. Their insistence on exclusive rights was undermined in the 16th and 17th centuries by being few in number, by their high cost, by their tendency to side with the Royalists in the Civil War and by their abandonment of London during the Great Plague.

Meanwhile, the surgeons' history differs markedly, reflecting their craft origins. Although surgery was carried out in medieval hospitals (p. 35), it could not be performed by those in Holy Orders. Given their dexterity with razors, barbers were called upon to operate under the direction of monks. The surgical knowledge they thus acquired spread to barbers outside the hospitals. In 1308 the Company of Barbers was formed. Competition with the small, rival organisation, the Fellowship of Surgeons, was resolved by the formation of a new livery company in 1540, the Company of Barber-Surgeons, an uneasy collaboration that was, nevertheless, sustained for 200 years.

Eventually, the surgeons sought independence and formed their own Company of Surgeons in 1745, with their Hall located only 400 m from Newgate prison, a legitimate source of bodies for dissection. It was not long before the Company needed more space, partly to house John Hunter's museum of anatomical specimens. In 1800 the Company moved to a house in Lincoln's Inn Fields and, of greater significance, received a charter to become the Royal College of Surgeons of London.

There were no additional royal colleges created until 1930, but 11 were then established in the following 66 years, including three non-medical ones. Although the origins of each medical college are unique, several evolved from specialist medical societies (p. 184) seeking greater autonomy for their members by breaking away from within one of the existing colleges. For example, the Obstetricians & Gynaecologists left the Royal College of Surgeons in 1930. The creation of others reflected new areas of medical practice, such as the radiologists in 1975. Like the two oldest colleges, their principal aims are to advance the science and practice of their specialty. This is achieved by controlling entry to the specialty through setting the curriculum and conducting examinations, by approving training posts and programmes, and by setting professional standards and encouraging continuing professional development.

Unlike the medical colleges, the first two non-medical colleges to gain royal approval, the Royal College of Nursing (1939) and Royal College of Midwives (1947), were responsible for protecting not only professional standards, but also terms and conditions of employment. The latter extended to affiliation with the Trades Unions Congress. The most recent addition has been the Royal College of Speech & Language Therapists in 1995.

the opposite side of the street on the corner with Mansfield Street. Since 1957 this has been the home of the **Royal College of Midwives**.

It was not until 1881 that female midwives organised themselves to meet the growing encroachment of man-midwives, as doctors practising obstetrics were known. Zepherina Veitch and Louisa Hubbard founded the Matron's Aid Society with the aim 'to raise the efficiency and improve the status of midwives and to petition parliament for their recognition'. They were joined in 1886 by Rosalind Paget. To raise their profile and clarify their role, the Society was renamed the Midwives Institute and Trained Nurses Club.

Their campaigning met resistance not only from doctors, who saw it as a threat to their livelihoods, but also from Ethel Bedford Fenwick of the British Nursing Council,

who resented the establishment of an alternative organisation to her own. Despite this, the campaign soon paid off when, in 1902, the Midwives' Act established the Central Midwives Board in England to govern training and regulate the profession, and made it illegal for unqualified midwives to practise. But their survival was not assured until the passing of the 1911 National Insurance Act, which protected the right of married women to chose between a doctor and a midwife during childbirth (p. 22).

The organisation was renamed the College of Midwives in 1941

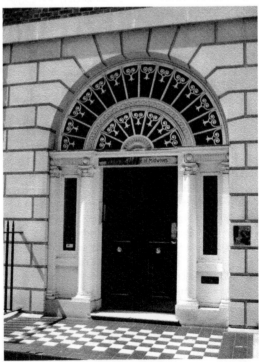

The Royal College of Midwives, with its iconic blue door, has been in Mansfield Street since 1957

and gained a Royal Charter in 1947. Although from its inception the organisation had worked to improve the status and rights of midwives, it was not until 1976 that it formally became a trade union. Like the Royal College of Nursing, it combines that role with a concern for professional standards.

Continue along New Cavendish Street until you reach Portland Place, one of the grandest thoroughfares in London, designed by Robert Adam in the 1770s. This was another favoured residence of doctors in the 19th century, although unlike Harley Street name plates were prohibited so they had to leave their visiting cards on display in the windows. The large building on the other side of New Cavendish Street on your right, No. 23, is the headquarters of the **Nursing & Midwifery Council**, the regulator of those professions. Although only established in 2002, this building was constructed in 1937 for the Nursing and Midwifery Council's predecessors, the General Nursing Council (1919–83) and the UK Central Council for Nurses, Midwives & Health Visitors (1983–2002). In the 1990s the regulator oversaw the most significant change in nursing since the early 20th century: the shift of nursing training from about 1,500 independent schools associated with hospitals to the universities. Training ceased to be largely an apprenticeship and became more like that for other health care professions.

Beyond it, No. 21, has been the home of the **Association of Anaesthetists** since 2002. Until 1900 there were only two royal colleges, physicians and surgeons, reflecting the traditional distinction between those who theorised about internal, invisible conditions (hence the American label, internal medicine) and empirics who tackled external, visible problems. Generally, the former had used drugs and the latter the knife. With the increasing complexity of medicine in the 20th century, doctors felt the need to form Associations (covering the British Isles) to enhance their public image, promote their specialist interests and 'promote friendship among practitioners'. They felt that such activities were not within the remit of existing professional bodies. The physicians formed an Association in 1907, followed by the surgeons in 1920, the paediatricians in 1928 and the anaesthetists in 1932.

Until about 1930 most anaesthetics were given by general practitioners who were poorly paid and dependent on surgeons for access to private patients. The Association of Anaesthetists successfully helped raise the standing of anaesthetists, which led to greater recognition within the Royal College of Surgeons and in 1992 to the creation of their own royal college. Despite such success, the Association continues as an independent voice promoting the development and interests of the specialty. Its home includes the Anaesthesia Heritage Centre, which documents the history of anaesthesia and is open to the public (www.aagbi.org).

Cross Portland Place and stop outside No. 36, the home of the **British Institute of Radiology**, an example of a specialist society. The

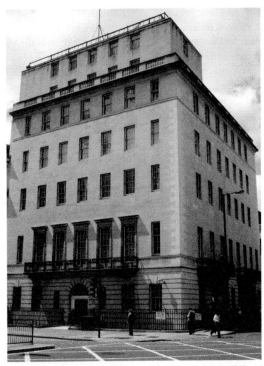

Built in 1937, this rather austere and somewhat Soviet-style building has been home to the nurses' (and since 1983, midwives' and health visitors') regulatory body. The fanlight above the door came from the 1776 Adam house that stood on this site

discovery of X-rays in 1895 led within a year to their use in diagnosis. The physicists and doctors involved formed the X-ray Society in 1897, which emerged in the 1920s as the British Institute of Radiology. As with the anaesthetists, from the 1930s medical radiologists together with radiotherapists sought professional recognition and autonomy, which culminated in the establishment of the **Royal College of Radiologists** in 1979. The college is based next door at No. 38. Like the other colleges formed in the 20th century,

it is largely dependent on members' subscriptions and the examination fees it can charge those seeking postgraduate diplomas. Despite the successful creation of a medical royal college, the multidisciplinary specialist society continues to thrive next door at No. 36.

Across the road you can just see No. 41 (it has a blue plaque), which, from 1947 to 2008, was the home of the **Novartis** (previously, Ciba) **Foundation** set up by a Swiss pharmaceutical company. Its particular contribution was to encourage links between scientists and clinicians from different backgrounds who would otherwise rarely meet and collaborate. Its international meetings and symposia often proved decisive in advancing knowledge and understanding. In 2010 it merged with the **Academy of Medical Sciences**, an organisation committed to promoting medical science and encouraging the adoption of scientific advances.

Continue along New Cavendish Street and turn left into Hallam Street. After 100 m, stop opposite No. 44, the home of the **General Medical Council** from 1922 to 2007. These custom-built premises, designed by Eustace Frere, have a fine bas-relief over the entrance showing medical practice at the time of Hippocrates. The Medical Act of 1858 required the establishment of a register of all recognised doctors and the standardisation of medical education, tasks for which the General Medical Council was created. The introduction of the register had the effect the doctors had hoped for, that of restricting access to only those who were 'properly' qualified. By the 1870s this had resulted in a shortage of practitioners, but doctors' income and status had been enhanced. The supremacy of allopathic (biomedical) practitioners had been established. And with the compulsory inclusion of midwifery in basic medical training, male

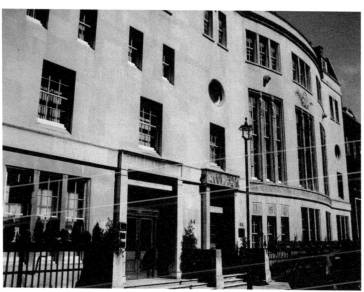

A fine pair of buildings designed by Eustace Frere in 1922, the right-hand one built for the General Medical Council, the left-hand one the original home of the Royal College of Paediatrics & Child Health up until 2008 but previously housing the Medical Protection Society

Walk 6

doctors had triumphed over female midwives. Despite a certain amount of public rhetoric, the interests of the public were always a secondary consideration for the profession in the 19th century.

Since 1900 most of the attention that the General Medical Council has attracted has arisen from its a role in policing the conduct of doctors. This has largely concerned sexual misconduct or drug abuse rather than poor clinical performance. Its tendency to protect doctors from patients, rather than the reverse, has in part reflected the composition of the Council, which until recently was dominated by doctors, although this has decreased from 94% in 1950 to 50% in 2012.

Next door, No. 50 was home to the youngest royal college, the **Royal College of Paediatrics & Child Health** from its formation in 1996

until 2008. Like the Royal College of Radiologists, it owes its existence to campaigning by an Association, the British Paediatric Association. Established in 1928 by a group of doctors specialising in the care of children, its spiritual home was the Old England Hotel, Windermere, where they regularly met until 1958.

This building, like that of its neighbour the General Medical Council, was constructed in 1922. From 1960 to 1997 it had been the home of the **Medical Protection Society**. At the end of the 19th century, doctors and dentists were taking action against an increasing number of unregistered and unqualified practitioners. In addition, a number of high-profile negligence and criminal cases, prompted by patients' accusations, made the headlines, and it was clear that individual doctors did not have

Medical profession

The creation of a single medical profession took many years to achieve. Until 1745 there were major differences between the three contenders as regards their backgrounds, training, social status, income and practice. Physicians were 'gentlemen', trained in classics and humanities at Oxbridge who then came to London for six months' hospital practice 'walking the wards'. They advised, rather than treated, patients about internal illnesses (still being known as internists in the USA). Few in number, only the rich could afford their services. A licence from the royal college (p. 194)

was needed to practise in and within seven miles of London.

In contrast, surgeons were empiricists, treating external problems such as abscesses and fractures, work that required speed and dexterity. Surgery was a craft for which training was by apprenticeship and, as for other crafts, the governing body was a City Company, the Barber-Surgeons.

Apothecaries were lower-middle-class tradesmen who officially were restricted to compounding and dispensing drugs. However, they were the only source of medical advice for many people, an activity formally recognised in 1704, although they were still only permitted to charge for the medicines they prescribed.

In 1745, to distinguish themselves from the barbers, the surgeons broke away and formed the Company of Surgeons. Similarly, apothecaries, recognising the need to develop a separate identity from dispensers, decided to exclude the latter from their governing body, the Society of Apothecaries, in 1774.

Despite continuing differences between the three occupations, they were united in their opposition to unlicensed practitioners. When the Medical Society of London was established in 1773, there were equal numbers of physicians, surgeons and apothecaries.

In 1800 the surgeons changed from a City Company to a royal college in recognition of their professional status. Of greater significance was the Apothecaries Act of 1815, which required that anyone wanting to be a general practitioner in London, apart from physicians, had to be licensed by Apothecaries' Hall. The Act, in effect, entrusted the examination of 75% of medical practitioners to the Society of Apothecaries.

By the mid-19th century, the distinctions between the three traditions were increasingly artificial. In reality, two categories had emerged with the growth of hospitals, general practitioners and consultants, a distinction that largely persists to the present day. By 1856, of the 10,000 licensed practitioners in England, 56% were surgeon-apothecaries, 19% were surgeons, 12% were apothecaries and only 4% were physicians.

Reform had been underway for some time before the 1858 Medical Act formally unified physicians, surgeons and apothecaries, recognised their equal status and granted them exclusive rights to practise medicine. It also introduced governmental control over medical education and the involvement of physicians in general medical training, although it was not until 1883 that the two royal colleges established the Conjoint Exam, which awarded a diploma (MRCS, LRCP) that granted entry to the newly unified medical profession. During the 20th century, universities became the main source of qualifications, although the Society of Apothecaries still provides a route into medicine through its United Examining Board.

the resources to defend themselves in these cases. The case that triggered action was when a Dr David Bradley was wrongly convicted of assaulting a woman in his surgery. He was later pardoned, but only after spending eight months in prison.

The need for strength in numbers was obvious, and a number of mutual medical defence organisations were started, the first national one being the Medical Defence Union in 1885. However, members' concerns about a lack of accountability and certain irregularities in its running led to a breakaway group in 1892 forming a rival, the Medical Protection Society. From the start, work focused on taking action to exclude 'quacks'. Members sometimes acted as bogus patients to entrap unlicensed practitioners, such as the vendor of a treatment to eradicate obesity and 'a gang of Hindoo oculists' who excised the 'skin' over the cornea. From funding the legal costs of its members, it expanded its role to paying for any compensation a doctor was required to pay to a patient. Nowadays it also takes a preventive approach, advising doctors and dentists about ethical aspects of clinical practice. Like other defence organisations, its role has changed since the introduction in 1990 of Crown Immunity (in which the state takes responsibility for the activities carried out in the NHS).

Continue along Hallam Street, cross Weymouth Street and turn right into Devonshire Street. Turn left into Great Portland Street, where you will pass, on your left after about 100 m, an example of just how large and sophisticated modern private hospitals have become compared with the nursing homes of the early 20th century. **The Portland Hospital** was purpose-built in 1983, specialising in the care of women and children. It has over 100 beds, four operating theatres and intensive care facilities. The other big change in private hospitals over the past century has been their ownership. Like most private hospitals, this one is owned by a huge corporation

that trades them like any other commodity. In this case, it is the Hospital Corporation of America, which had a worldwide turnover of about $30 billion in 2010.

On the opposite side of the street (No. 234) is another example of the transfer of property between the public and private sectors. The old **Royal National Orthopaedic Hospital**, built in 1905, now houses the outpatient facilities for the Portland Hospital.

At the end of Great Portland Street, cross Euston Road and turn left along the front of the small elegant Albany Terrace. Turn right into Park Square East which takes you into Regent's Park. After 100 m you will see to the right one of the finest modernist buildings in London, the **Royal College of Physicians**. The college was founded in 1518 by a group led by Thomas Linacre, their aim being to protect the interests of Oxbridge-educated physicians by gaining control of the exclusive right to practise medicine. In the event, protection only covered the City of London and a seven-mile radius. Despite this early success, battles with the surgeons and apothecaries (both City livery companies rather than colleges) continued until the 19th century. The claim of the physicians for exclusivity failed because they were few in number and their high cost meant few people had access to them. Their case was further weakened by the decision of most to side with the Royalists in the Civil War (1640s) and their abandonment of London during the Great Plague (1665).

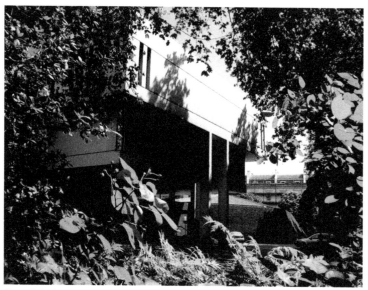

One of the finest modernist buildings in London, Denys Lasdun's Royal College of Physicians, built in 1963

The College of Physicians was initially located in the City. As medical London shifted west in the 19th century so did the college, first to a new home in Trafalgar Square and then to here in 1964. Rather than orient the building towards Regent's Park, the modernist architect, Denys Lasdun, had the main windows look to the right, over the college garden and the Georgian houses of St Andrew's Terrace. The latter were acquired in the 1980s for extra accommodation. Step inside the main building to see the spacious hall or atrium with a central staircase that takes your eyes up towards the portraits of past Presidents, the more distant of whom would probably be perplexed by the range of modern-day practitioners and the complexity of managing the professions.

Retrace your steps to Great Portland Street underground station on Euston Road, where the walk ends.

Walk 6

Walk 7: 'Merrie Islington' to 'the contagion of numbers'

Although hospitals have dominated health care over the past 250 years, the vast majority of care throughout history has been provided in or near people's homes. Primary health care, provided locally by generalists (rather than specialists), meeting common everyday needs and being directly available has always existed, even if its appearance has changed over time. This walk is a journey through four eras of primary health care.

During the first era (before 1780), the prevailing explanation of death and disease was that they were caused by imbalances in the four humours (key fluids) of the body – blood, choler (yellow bile), phlegm and black bile. All manner of practitioners claimed to be able to restore balance, and thus health. While wealth afforded a visit from a university-educated physician or the services of a surgeon, most people had to make do with medications dispensed by an apothecary, chemist or druggist. Otherwise there were lay carers (relatives, neighbours, friends) or all manner of unlicensed practitioners. An alternative was to put your faith in the increasing number of spas, whose owners made bold claims for the healing powers of their waters. As you will see, this area of London boasted several such establishments.

During the second era, which lasted until about 1900, London was breaking out of its traditional confines and spreading up through the fields of Finsbury to Islington and beyond. With agriculture in crisis, people flocked to the metropolis in the hope of work, bewitched by what the social investigator Hubert

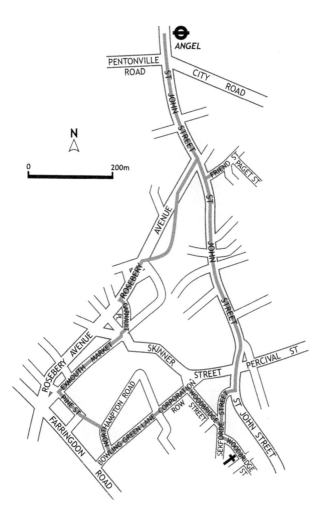

Llewellyn-Smith called 'the contagion of numbers'. The population of Finsbury grew from 55,000 in 1801 to 129,000 in 1861, and that of Islington from 10,000 to 155,000. Subsequently, those who could afford it moved further out to the suburbs as railway and tram systems provided cheap and quick access. However, far from the population in Finsbury and Islington decreasing, many of the vacated homes were divided up, and population density increased. Islington reached 335,000 in number by the end of the 19th century. Urbanisation and industrialisation brought with them a growing underclass of paupers, suffering poor health.

The level of poverty concerned many of the more fortunate, who were benefiting from London's economic success. Private philanthropy led to the establishment of voluntary dispensaries: one was established in Finsbury in 1780 and one in Islington in 1821. Throughout both this and the earlier era, people could also seek advice and treatment from chemists and druggists, two trades that merged in 1815 and redefined themselves as 'pharmacists' in the 1840s. They continue today to make an important contribution to primary care.

Increasing concern that people who were not impoverished were abusing the charity of voluntary dispensaries, plus the need to raise funds by charging patients a small amount, led to the establishment of social insurance schemes run by Friendly Societies (self-help groups of workers), churches and other organisations. Another option was to pay a small amount each week directly to a provident dispensary to cover the cost of care when they fell ill. And for the underclass of paupers, the parishes made some very limited provision through the Poor Law. Those not forced by Poor Law Guardians to enter the workhouse received outdoor relief (equivalent to modern-day social security payments). From 1873 some Poor Law Unions (groups of parishes) established Poor Law Dispensaries.

The third era, which started about 1900, reflected the growing acceptance that the health care system was neither sustainable financially nor adequate in meeting most people's needs. Biomedical views of the causes of disease, its investigation and its treatment were about to take a great leap forward. While most of the attention was focused on the need to coordinate and plan hospitals, primary care was not ignored. Small voluntary social insurance schemes were proving inadequate, and in 1911 Lloyd George introduced compulsory National Health Insurance in which the state accepted responsibility for ensuring that all manual and low-paid non-manual workers had access to designated general practitioners (so-called 'panel' doctors) by contributing 5 pence for every 4 pence contributed by workers. Despite this, the need for charity persisted as the scheme did not cover dependants and the unemployed. This meant a continuing role not only for the voluntary dispensaries, but also for the medical missions that had been established by churches in the late 19th century.

In addition, during the early 20th century, voluntary organisations established clinics for those whose needs were barely being met: infant welfare; maternity care; family planning; and massage (physiotherapy) for soldiers injured during World War I. Despite visionary proposals in the 1920s to build modern health centres, only two materialised in London before World War II. However, recognition by parliament of the state's responsibilities resulted in the establishment of municipal clinics for infant welfare in 1918 and later for tuberculosis and for family planning.

The fourth era dates from the start of the NHS in 1948. Finally, services could be coordinated and planned. At least in theory. In practice, another attempt to introduce health centres was thwarted by the GPs, who refused to relinquish their independence. As a result, dependence on hospitals was extended for another half-century, the development of primary care was set back, and the public had to put up with the vagaries of lone practitioners in inadequate premises. However, in recent years, some progress has been made, with custom-built premises for multiprofessional health care teams appearing. Throughout all these changes, alternative or complementary healers have, with mixed success, continued to offer their services.

Apart from the history of primary care, this walk also illustrates the way in which crowded urban populations depend on their rural hinterland. As early as the 16th century, Stow had described Islington as:

> 'a place of fields commodius for citizens therein to walke, shoote and otherwise to recreate and refresh their dulled spirits in the sweete and wholesome ayre.'

Until 1800 inhabitants of the crowded City depended on 'merrie Islington' for fresh air and 'medicinal' waters to maintain and restore their health, while its almshouses provided sanctuary for the old and infirm, and its private madhouses provided seclusion and respite for those deemed to be mentally ill. It even provided temporary accommodation for those being inoculated against smallpox. Little wonder that Islington was described as 'London hospital'.

All this was to change over the following 150 years as urban development escaped the confines of the City and rolled out across the fields of Finsbury and up the hill to Islington. With that as a backdrop, you can start your journey, back in 1700.

The walk starts at Angel underground station. On leaving the station, turn left along Islington High Street and after 50 m, at the traffic lights, cross over into St John Street and onto the far side of the road.

In 1700 simple buildings lined both sides of the road. On the other side, you would have seen **Owen's Almshouses** (similar to modern-day sheltered housing for the elderly). Almshouses were established either by City Guilds/Companies or by philanthropic individuals, such as these, paid for by Alice Owen (but bequeathed to the Worshipful Company of Brewers). Often there would be a resident nurse or supervisor, enabling infirm people to maintain their independence. The alternative prospect after a lifetime's hard labour for those with no family support was the parish workhouse. The ten houses survived until 1840 when they were rebuilt about 100 m further along on the left. These, in turn, were demolished in 1879.

After 100 m, cross Rosebery Avenue and walk along it 50 m as far as the gate to Spa Green, a small park. The hillside that you see stretching down towards modern-day Clerkenwell was full of natural chalybeate springs (impregnated with iron), which, in the 17th and 18th centuries, were believed to have medicinal properties. Several springs had been known about before the Reformation by the priests of the Priory of Clerkenwell but remained hidden until, in 1683, Thomas Sadler

Walk 7

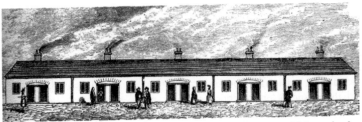

Almshouses established in St John Street by Alice Owen in 1611, which survived until 1840 when they were rebuilt nearby

rediscovered one in the grounds of the Musick House he had just opened (on the site of the present-day theatre). Sadler's Wells provided not only health-giving water (p. 259) but also entertainment. A theatre has occupied this site continuously ever since.

Enter Spa Green and walk through the park. This was the site of **Islington Spa**, also known in the 18th century as New Tunbridge Wells, due to the similar composition of its water to that of the then fashionable spa in Kent. It sought to emulate the latter, providing a low-cost alternative much closer to London. The waters were seen as both curative and preventive, helpful for mental as well as physical health. The power of the water was not doubted by those promoting it, who claimed it could 'cure of the Jaundice, Nervous, and all other Weaknesses, Fluxes of Blood of every kind, Gravel, &c.'. There was a lodging house where invalids could receive bed and board. For the poor, the charge for the standard half-pint of water was waived if you were referred by a doctor. The spa, which

functioned from May to October, was considerably more than just an elaborate spring – additional diversions included tree-lined walks, a bowling green, a dance hall, a coffee house or breakfast room (40 feet long, with an orchestra), raffles and even lectures. Despite its somewhat humble origins, by the 1720s it had become a fashionable resort of the aristocracy, particularly for breakfasting, even attracting the daughters of George II, who were, apparently, as coarse as any Hanoverians, with a taste for crude jokes, horses and their grooms.

By the 1790s the Spa was in decline. London's population was starting to expand exponentially, a trend that was to continue for the next 200 years. The fields between where you are standing and the City of London to the south were built on during the 19th century, mostly with terraced houses and small industrial works. Some buildings from that period survive, although many suffered bomb damage during World War II and others were demolished after the war to make way for modern, often high-rise, homes and offices.

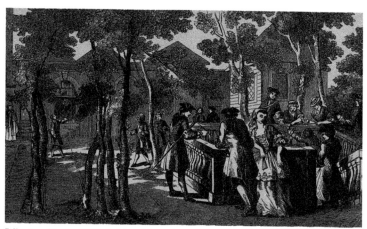

Islington Spa in 1737, fashionable and popular as much for the social opportunities it offered as for any medicinal benefits

Leave Spa Green by the gate at the end and continue straight on along Green Terrace. After about 50 m bear left along Garnault Place, at the end of which bear right along Exmouth Market. At the end turn left into Pine Street, where, about 50 m on the left, you will see a **Maternity & Child Welfare Centre** built in 1927. Around 1900 it was realised and accepted that health care was partly the responsibility of government and the state. It was also recognised that attempts had to be made to prevent disease rather than waiting until people fell ill. Initially, it was up to each local authority to decide what action to take. However, by 1917 only about 400 infant welfare centres (in which nurses carried out screening, developmental monitoring, surveillance, health education, and antenatal care) had been established in the whole of Britain. So, in 1918 the Maternity and Child Welfare Act was passed,

which required local authorities to establish services for mothers and infants. One consequence was that the Medical Officers of Health, who were responsible, introduced doctors, who largely took over the services from nurses. By 1948 local authorities in Britain ran 4,700 such clinics. Over time, these services were incorporated into mainstream general practice, negating the need for special clinics. Reflecting demographic changes, the building is now a day centre for the elderly. An original gas-light fitting can be seen on the front right corner.

Continue into Catherine Griffiths Court, where you will see the **Finsbury Health Centre**. In the 19th and early 20th centuries, Finsbury consisted of streets of overcrowded terraced houses in which poor sanitation and smog encouraged disease. In the 1920s government concern about the poor state of primary care (p. 211) led

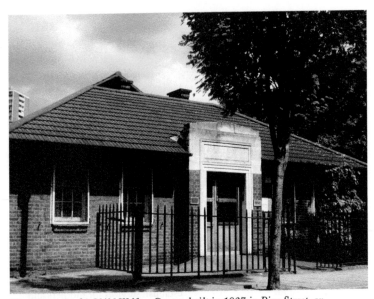

The Maternity & Child Welfare Centre, built in 1927 in Pine Street, an example of the involvement of local government in health care following an Act of Parliament in 1918

to the commissioning of a wide-ranging review. The result was the visionary Dawson Report, which proposed health centres as the basis of a comprehensive, hierarchical health care system. Dismissed by the government, the vision was kept alive by, among others, the Socialist Medical Association, which was influenced by the successes of the Soviet polyclinics. Thanks to two local councils in London, the dream was realised in the 1930s when two contrasting health centres were built: Peckham Health Centre focused on preventing disease and promoting health, whereas Finsbury was seen as less ambitious (although perhaps more realistic in that it has survived) in aiming to treat established disease.

The Finsbury Plan adopted by the socialist council in the 1930s envisaged a health centre alongside public baths, libraries and nurseries (although only the health centre was ever built). It was the first municipal commission of a modernist building in the UK, designed by Berthold Lubetkin and the Tecton Group. Following his philosophy that 'Nothing is too good for ordinary people', Lubetkin created a building more akin to a club or drop-in centre. In attempting to create a relaxed, welcoming atmosphere, he had no formal reception desk (although one was later installed). There were murals encouraging exposure to fresh air and sunlight, and the use of glass bricks to create

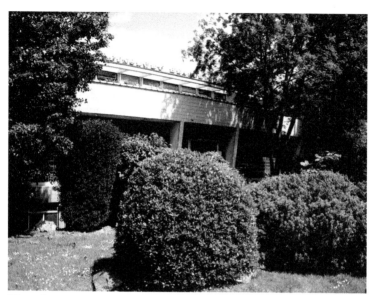

The radical Finsbury Health Centre designed by Berthold Lubetkin and the Tecton Group in 1938, the first modernist building commissioned by local government in Britain

a light airy environment. Alongside general practitioners were a TB clinic, chiropody, dentistry and a solarium. And the whole design was flexible to meet anticipated changes in health care technology.

Primary care

Although hospitals have dominated health care over the past 250 years, the vast majority of care has been provided in or near people's homes. Primary health care, provided locally, by generalists (rather than specialists), meeting common needs and being directly available (without the need for referral) to the public has always existed, even if its appearance has changed.

Before 1780 the prevailing explanation of disease was imbalances in the four humours (key fluids) of the body. All manner of practitioners claimed to be able to restore balance, and thus health. While the wealthy were visited by a university-educated physician, most people had to make do with lay carers (relatives, neighbours, friends) or a multitude of unlicensed practitioners. As an alternative, there were 'medicinal' spas, whose owners made dramatic claims for the healing powers of their water (p. 259).

From the late 18th century, there was increasing concern about the lack of health care for the poor. Those prepared to undergo means testing and risk incarceration in a workhouse could get limited help under the Poor Law. But the majority were dependent on the outpatient departments of voluntary general hospitals or dispensaries. However, increasing concern that people were abusing the charity of such establishments led to the creation of provident dispensaries and of insurance schemes run by Friendly Societies (self-help groups of workers), which, through a regular contribution, gave them access to the 'club doctor'. The latter covered about one third of adult workers but not their dependants.

By 1900 dependence on voluntary contributions was proving inadequate and was replaced in 1911 by National Health Insurance (compulsory for all manual and low-paid non-manual workers), in which the state more than matched the individual's contribution – '9 pence for 4 pence'. Fifteen million people now had access to any doctors who participated ('the panel'). However, the need for charity persisted as the scheme did not cover people's dependants or the unemployed. This meant a continuing role not only for the voluntary dispensaries, but also for the medical missions that had been established by the churches. Meanwhile, private charities established services such as family planning and physiotherapy, responsibilities eventually taken on by local government in 1930.

Despite visionary proposals in the 1920s for local government to establish health centres, only two materialised in London before World War II (Finsbury, Peckham). By 1942 half the population benefited from National Insurance. Most GPs had joined the 'panel,' although some survived purely on private patients. However, it was not until the start of the NHS in 1948 that universal access to primary care, irrespective of income or social status, was achieved. In theory, services could now be coordinated and planned. In practice, the introduction of health centres was still thwarted by the GPs, who refused to relinquish their independence. As a result, dependence on hospitals was extended for another half-century, with the development of custom-built premises for multiprofessional primary care teams a slow, tortuous process.

Despite the excitement and success surrounding Finsbury and Peckham health centres, no more were built before World War II. And after the war, Aneurin Bevan, the Minister of Health, failed to persuade GPs of the merits of health centres, which they saw as a threat to their independence. Bevan's forced abandonment of the policy increased the public's dependence on hospitals and inhibited the development of primary care for several decades. The outcome no doubt pleased Winston Churchill, who, in 1943, had banned a poster showing a shining Finsbury Health Centre against a picture of a starving rickety child in a slum with the slogan 'Your Britain – Fight for it Now'. He rejected the notion that the country was fighting for a socialist future (although the official reason for the ban was that he considered that rickets did not exist in London).

Continue on through Catherine Griffiths Court, along Northampton Road, and after 30 m turn left along Bowling Green Lane (a reminder of 17th century entertainments). After 100 m it becomes Corporation Row, and after another 100 m turn right into Woodbridge Street and stop outside No. 16, known in the 19th century as Woodbridge House.

In 1800, while the affluent were treated in their own homes by visiting doctors, the only way the working poor of London could consult a medical practitioner was either in a hospital outpatient department or at one of the recently established dispensaries (p. 229). At that time, specially designed buildings for providing health care were limited to a few of the voluntary hospitals. Most health care was provided in residential property such as Woodbridge House. From 1848 to 1871 this was the home of the **Finsbury Dispensary**, which had been established in 1780. It had moved five times, seeking ever-larger properties in which to expand its services.

The Finsbury Dispensary was the sixth to be established in London. Its organisation and activities followed a common plan, chiefly the work of one of London's leading physicians, John Coakley Lettsom.

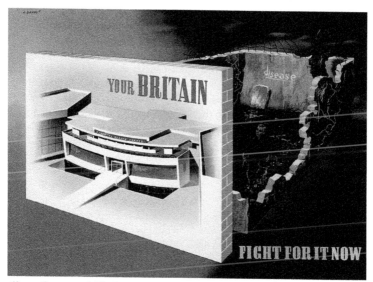

Abram Games used Finsbury Health Centre as a symbol of the better future being fought for in a propaganda poster supporting the war effort in the 1940s

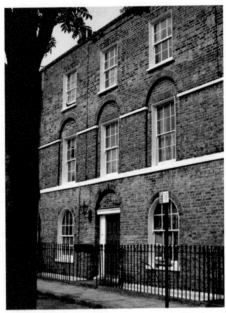

Woodbridge House was, from 1848 to 1971, home to the Finsbury Dispensary, one of the earliest voluntary dispensaries established in London

Their establishment depended on the support of a group of local, concerned citizens who were prepared to subscribe money. In the case of Finsbury, the leading light was George Friend, who had made his money as a dyer of cloth with the East India Company. In return for a donation, subscribers were entitled to provide access (recommendations) to free care for members of 'the labouring and necessitous poor'. The extent of each subscriber's entitlement related directly to the amount of money donated each year – in 1845, each was 'entitled annually to fifteen General Letters of Recommendation for every Guinea subscribed'. The support of royalty, even foreign royalty, was an asset as

it helped to attract other subscribers. For some unknown reason, the Belgian monarch supported the dispensary from 1831 onwards, support that even included a visit in 1937 by the reigning monarch, King Leopold. To encourage donations, fund-raising dinners and festivals were held, and local churches donated one Sunday collection each year. The dispensary even benefited from John Wesley preaching a sermon in its support in 1788.

Finsbury Dispensary was fairly typical in employing a resident apothecary and having several part-time physicians and surgeons (one of whom attended every day except Sundays), some paid, others honorary. It served an extensive area from Holborn in the south to Pentonville in the north, and from Grays Inn Road in the west to City Road in the east. As the population of this area grew rapidly, so did the need for health care for the poor. In 1871 the dispensary moved to custom-built premises on a site near the Angel that you will visit later.

Continue along Woodbridge Street, crossing Sekforde Street, and after 30 m stop outside Woodbridge Chapel. This was built in 1832, and from 1945 to 1995 the chapel and the neighbouring house, No. 5, were the home of the **Clerkenwell Medical Mission**. Medical missions were established in London from 1871 onwards to provide free health care to impoverished, destitute people who could not gain access to

a voluntary dispensary but wanted to avoid the workhouse. The staff were as committed to providing spiritual salvation as to treating physical illness. They were aware that people were more susceptible to a religious message when in need of help for their health, in the same way that health care staff today take the opportunity to proselytise about health-promoting lifestyles when people are ill.

This mission started life in 1889 as Islington Medical Mission (you will see its previous homes later) and moved here in 1945. For 50 years general practitioners ran a surgery on the first floor of No. 5. Although the NHS took over paying the doctor in 1948, all other costs continued to be met by the mission. Services

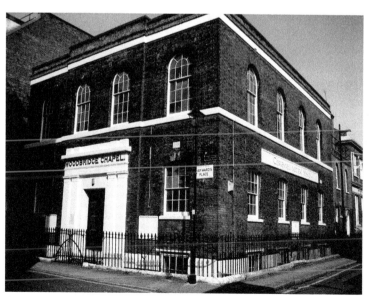

Clerkenwell Medical Mission provided primary care and social welfare services in Woodbridge Chapel and in the adjoining house (far right) from 1945 to 1995

Walk 7

included dentistry and an eye clinic, both of which were provided in cubicles in the side aisles of the adjoining chapel (which survive). In addition, staff provided free clothing, toys and hot lunches. The mission closed in 1995 when they were unable to recruit a new doctor, given the small number of registered patients that remained.

Retrace your steps along Woodbridge Street and bear right up Sekforde Street, largely untouched since its construction in the late 18th century. At the end, turn left along St John Street and stop after about 150 m, opposite Wycliff Street. The 19th century yellow-brick building on the right-hand side of Wycliff Street was the site of **Northampton Manor House**. Up until 1800 there were very limited public services for those suffering from mental illness

(p. 66). This had led to the growth of privately owned madhouses that varied in size from two or three patients to several hundred. One of the first to be established, in 1678, was in the old Northampton Manor House. By 1710 it was being run by James Newton, a herbalist, who created a botanic garden in the grounds to support his work. The gateway to the property was surmounted by figures of mad people with the promise of 'no cure, no money'.

Those deemed 'mad' could not always rely on friends and family. Once admitted, people were in danger of being abandoned, regardless of their social standing. This seems to have happened to Lady Mary Sattacoff, who entered Northampton Manor House on 21 November 1728. Two years later,

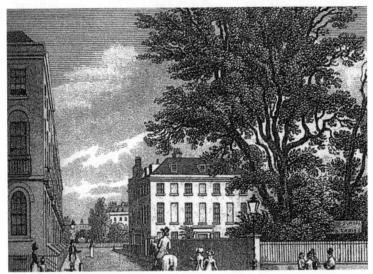

One of the first private madhouses to be established in London was Northampton Manor House in 1678

James Newton appealed in the Daily Post for:

> 'her sister, Prudence Bates, who for several months has not come to see her sister ... neither have sent her any conveniences, or clothes of any kind, nor payment for her medicines, or entertainment for this past year ... Whoever discovers the said Mrs Prudence Bates that she may be brought to justice and convicted of the said fraud shall receive two guineas from me.'

Concern about the terrible conditions in many private madhouses and the circumstances by which people were admitted grew during the 18th century. In 1763 the *Gentleman's Magazine* drew attention to the fact that people who were quite sane were frequently lodged in madhouses by relatives who wanted them out of the way. A man might send his wife to one because she was 'extravagant', and daughters were admitted in order to break off romances that their families disapproved of.

Following Newton's death in the 1750s, the house was under the control of William Battie, who was also the first physician of the newly established St Luke's Hospital for Lunatics in Moorfields. Northampton Manor House ceased to be a madhouse in 1803, becoming a ladies' boarding school before being demolished in 1869.

Continue along St John Street and stop on the corner of the next street on the left, Whiskin Street. This used to be a street of terraced houses, in one of which a **New Tuberculosis Dispensary** was established. Tuberculosis (p. 218) (also known as phthisis or consumption) was a major cause of illness and death until the middle of the 20th century. Although a Phthisical Dispensary had been established in Chancery Lane as early as 1805, it, like others created in the 19th century, focused solely on treating the patient rather than also trying to stop the spread of the disease. Following the discovery in 1882 of the bacterium that causes tuberculosis, a new approach was advocated in which not only was the disease treated, but also the sufferer was taught how to avoid infecting others. In addition, active efforts were made to find 'unknown' cases in the community. The first TB dispensary committed to this approach in London was established in Paddington in 1909. With government encouragement, local authorities set up similar dispensaries, although the one here in Whiskin Street was not established until 1931.

Another area of responsibility taken on by local authorities around that time was birth control. Continue up St John Street, cross to the other side at the next junction and stop on the corner of Spencer Street by the cattle trough. This street is now lined with university buildings that replaced terraces of fine Georgian townhouses. In one of them, the **Goswell Women's Welfare Clinic** was established in 1936. Although Marie Stopes had established the first family planning clinic in the

Walk 7

Tuberculosis

Tuberculosis (phthisis, scrofula, consumption) was a major cause of illness and death until the middle of the 20th century. It was spread both through the air from person to person and by milk from infected cows. From Henry I (1100–1135) onwards, English monarchs claimed divine healing powers for the King's Evil, as TB was known. The ceremony was formal, with the King touching the sufferer's throat while a cleric intoned 'They shall lay their hands on the sick and they shall recover'. Some monarchs (James I, William III) discontinued the practice, only for others to restore it. The last to 'lay on hands' was Queen Anne in 1712, although in France the practice continued until the revolution in 1789.

Belief in the benefits of fresh air and sea-water led to the establishment of many coastal institutions, the most famous being the Royal Sea Bathing Hospital at Margate in 1791. Meanwhile in London, the first specialist service was the Phthisical Dispensary, set up in Chancery Lane in 1805. The first voluntary specialist hospital (p. 119) was founded in 1814 by a doctor, Isaac Buxton, as the Infirmary for Asthma, Consumption and other Pulmonary Diseases in Spitalfields. In 1849 it moved to City Road as the Royal Hospital for Diseases of the Chest. Meanwhile two other chest hospitals had been established in London – the Hospital for Consumption and Diseases of the Chest in Fulham (1842) and the City of London Hospital for Diseases

of the Chest in Spitalfields (1848), which moved to Hackney in 1855. Another was added in 1859, the North London Hospital for Consumption in Hampstead (later to become Mount Vernon Hospital).

The mainstay of treatment was fresh air and good nutrition. The former was clearly in short supply within London, so from the late 19th century the Metropolitan Asylums Board (p. 179) established sanatoria outside the city, mainly by converting existing buildings. Long periods of bed rest (often out of doors) remained the principal approach to treatment until the advent of effective drugs in the 1940s.

Meanwhile, following the discovery in 1882 by Robert Koch of the bacterium that causes tuberculosis (tubercle bacillus), Robert Philip, an Edinburgh doctor, advocated not only treating the disease, but also detecting early cases and preventing its spread. Philip's ideas caught on, and in 1909 the first TB dispensary in London to adopt his vision opened in Paddington. Implementation was helped in 1912 when a government committee recommended that Philip's system be copied all over the UK, with local authorities required to give free treatment to TB patients. The creation of TB dispensaries reflected a change in clinical policy from relying entirely on the incarceration of established cases in sanatoria, although such isolation may have contributed much to the eventually control of TB.

UK in 1921, there were still only four clinics in London a decade later. These were organised by the National Birth Control Council (later to become the Family Planning Association). Birth control was not seen as a legitimate component of health care, and much of the medical profession was opposed to such clinics. However, once the Ministry of Health gave local authorities permission to provide such services, dozens were established, including this one. Women paid one shilling (5 p) for their first visit and had to purchase their own appliances (such as caps). A special fund provided help for those in extreme poverty.

Continue on up St John Street and, after 200 m, turn right into Friend Street and stop outside Nos 1–3, on the left. From 1871 to 1950 the **Finsbury Dispensary** was located on this site in custom-built premises, New Dispensary House. While it was a fine building, the architect was conscious of the dispensary's charitable status and constrained finances, and ensured that 'no money whatever was laid out in useless decorations'.

Demand had reached about 25,000 consultations a year by the time the dispensary moved here from the house in Woodbridge Street you have already seen. And it continued to grow, peaking at over 41,000 a

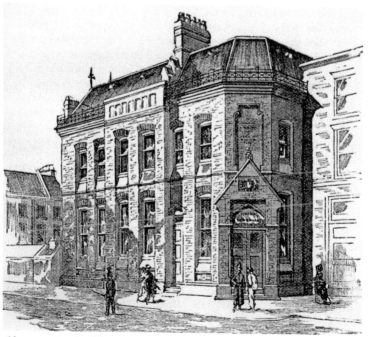

After occupying six different houses between 1780 and 1871, Finsbury Dispensary finally acquired its own custom-built premises, New Dispensary House, which functioned until World War II bombing destroyed it

Walk 7

year in the 1890s. This was partly because it was by then attracting patients from as far as Hoxton, Shoreditch and Haggerston. The vast majority were suffering from infectious diseases, including smallpox, diarrhoea, typhoid, whooping cough and tuberculosis.

Up until it moved here, free care had been provided (although a letter of recommendation was needed). But the steadily increasing demands on the budget led to the introduction of a patient fee (or co-payment) of one penny for every 'parcel of medicine'. Subscribers believed this would not only raise funds but also have 'a further beneficial effect, in causing patients to feel that they are in some measure paying for the benefits they receive. It also places a check upon those who might be inclined to apply for medicine, though not really in want of it.' Demand subsequently declined, although this was partly due to a fall in the population of Finsbury (from 120,000 in the 1880s to 70,000 in the 1930s) and partly due to the start of National Insurance in 1911, which gave those in manual and low-paid non-manual employment access to private general practitioners ('panel' doctors).

By the 1930s local authority provision of primary care had started (such as Finsbury Health Centre and the specialised clinics for TB, mothers and infants, and family planning). The dispensary needed to modernise to survive. Services were expanded with the addition of a foot clinic employing a chiropodist and masseuse. It one regard at least it was ahead of its time: it introduced a job-share for two women doctors.

The onset of World War II saw the evacuation of women and children (who constituted the majority of patients) from central London. In addition, New Dispensary House was severely damaged by enemy bombing. Following the war, the establishment of NHS services meant that in theory no one needed the dispensaries (which were not incorporated into the NHS). Despite this, along with some other long-established dispensaries, it continued to provide care to a declining number of elderly people until it finally closed in 1961.

The only reminder of the dispensary's illustrious 181-year existence are the local street names: Friend Street named after the principal founder, and Paget Street named after Sir James Paget, a surgeon to the dispensary and the founder of pathology as a science. Return to St John Street, turn right and return to the Angel underground station (400 m).

Continue along Upper Street towards Islington Green (400 m), where you should take the right fork that leads into Essex Road. Stop after 200 m, on the corner of Queen's Head Street. The small block of flats you have just passed was the site of one of four sets of almshouses established in this area from the 16th century onwards, although only one has survived, which you will see in a few minutes. Continue along Essex Road, turn right into Queen's Head Street, and

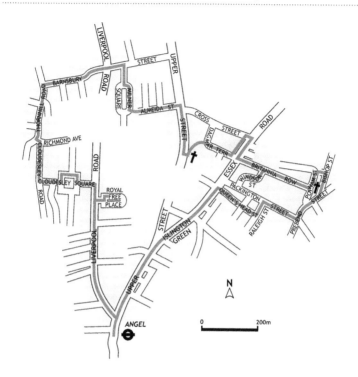

stop after about 30 m. This is where two more of the almshouses were sited. Those on the left side were founded by John Heath in 1640 for 'ten decayed members of the Company of Clothworkers, who receive annually a suit of clothes, a chaldron of coal (36 bushels or about 2 cubic yards) and £20'. They survived until the mid-19th century. Opposite, Jane Davis founded eight almshouses in 1794 with £2,000 left by her husband, a local carpenter. They housed married couples or widows aged 50 or more, who had to be Anglicans. She stipulated that no physician, surgeon or apothecary was to be a trustee as she suspected they might

not be able to resist 'using' the residents to develop their medical theories and interventions!

Walk on to the end of Queen's Head Street, turn left (Cruden Street), and then right into Packington Street. At the end, turn left into Prebend Street. Take the second street on the left (Bishop Street), which runs along the right hand side of the church. Beyond the church are the **Clothworkers' Almshouses**, the only surviving ones in the area, established in 1538 by Lady Margaret, Countess of Kent, and rebuilt in 1852. They continue to provide accommodation for eight women who also receive one cloak and a chaldron of coal

Walk 7

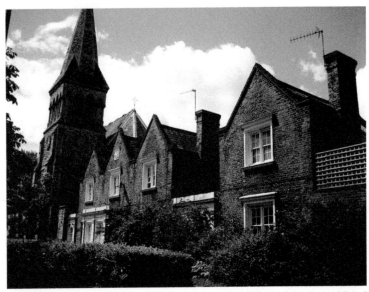

These Clothworkers' Almshouses, built in 1852, replaced those originally established on this site by the Countess of Kent in 1538

each year. You can see the arms of the clothworkers' guild on the eastern and northern sides of the buildings.

Walk round the almshouses and, as you approach the church, turn right along Britannia Row. Most of the 19th century terraced houses that lined the road were destroyed by a bomb in 1940. One of them had housed an **Almeric Paget Massage Clinic**, another example of a specialised primary care service that emerged during the 1930s. It is also an example of how independent individuals and organisations have introduced innovations into health care.

Recognising the rehabilitation needs of soldiers from World War I with muscular wounds, Almeric Paget and his wife decided in August 1914 to fund and provide

50 fully trained masseuses to provide massage, hydrotherapy and electrotherapy in the principal military hospitals in the UK. Thus began the Almeric Paget Massage Corps, which eventually numbered over 3,000. In November 1914 they established their first Massage and Electrical Out-Patient Clinic in London, with more clinics being established after the war. The one here in Britannia Row was not set up until 1931. The fact that by then Almeric Paget, who had become Baron Queenborough, was a Nazi sympathiser seemed to cause no difficulties, not even for Guy's Hospital where he was a governor.

After 100 m, turn left into Windsor Street, and about 50 m on the right, at a bend in the road, stop outside No. 13. This was the site of the initial home of the **Islington Medical Mission**, which, as you have seen, later became the Clerkenwell Medical Mission. Founded in 1890 by the Congregational Church, its contribution was as great as that of the long-established voluntary dispensaries. It had one resident and five visiting doctors plus a dentist, ten nurses and a dispenser.

Seeking more space, the Mission moved to the Congregational Church in Britannia Row in 1928, but, as you have just seen, most of the street was destroyed in 1940. The Mission found temporary accommodation locally during the war years but,

in 1945, the offer of space at Woodbridge Chapel in Clerkenwell was too good an opportunity to turn down. However, the medical superintendent Dr Thomson chose to stay and maintain a medical presence in this area. He established the Islington Medical Centre in the former Islington Dispensary building on Upper Street (which you will see shortly); this functioned successfully until 1981 when a lack of new patients led to its closure.

Return to Britannia Row, turn left, and on reaching Essex Road turn right. After about 50 m, stop outside No. 78. In the late 19th century, this housed an example of

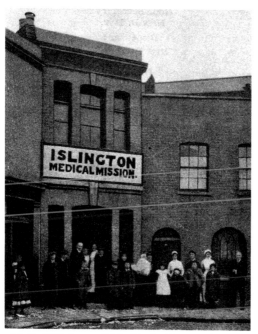

The Islington Medical Mission, established by the Congregational Church here in Windsor Street in 1890, provided primary care and social welfare for the most destitute and impoverished

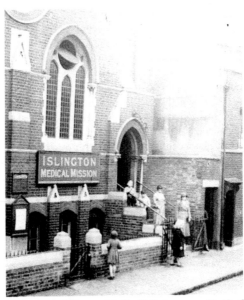

In search of more space, the Islington Medical Mission moved to the Congregational Church in Britannia Row in 1928

another key contributor to primary care provision, pharmacists (p. 225). You can see some remnants of **JTW Wallis's Patent Medicine & Drug Stores**: part of an advertisement for a treatment for catarrh still appears on the side wall, as does the iron bracket that would have held a large coloured lamp (a characteristic of pharmacies) over the side window.

Continue along Essex Road to the traffic lights and cross over to the raised pavement. If you look back diagonally across the traffic lights to the buildings beyond the small side street, you will see a short block of buildings with ground-floor shops. These stand on the site of **Fisher House**, a private madhouse in the 18th and 19th centuries. Its

most famous patient was Mary Lamb, the 'literary lunatic', who, together with her brother Charles, was a friend and fellow traveller of the Wordsworths, Coleridge and other 'romantics'. In 1796, under increasing family stress, Mary murdered her mother. The coroner declared her mad, but, in an unusually liberal act, placed her under the care of her brother rather than incarcerating her in Royal Bethlem Hospital (where people could be abandoned for life). She was immediately admitted to Fisher House, where Jess Annandale, the proprietor, apparently treated her affectionately.

For the rest of her life, Mary spent several months a year confined in madhouses during her periods

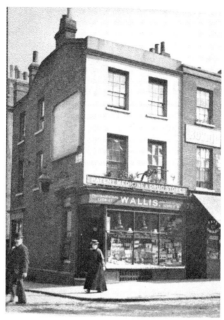

JTW Wallis's Patent Medicine & Drug Stores, photographed in 1895 by the owner's son, Charlie

Pharmacists

Chemists (dealers in chemicals) and druggists (who dealt in drugs of animal and vegetable origin) gradually merged during the 18th century, a development that was formally recognised by an Act of Parliament in 1815 that established their right to buy, compound, dispense and sell drugs and medicines. They were joined by those apothecaries who had chosen to focus on dispensing rather than giving medical advice, who, as members of the Society of Apothecaries, were part of the emerging medical profession (p. 200).

Until the 1840s chemists and druggists were essentially tradesmen, trained by apprenticeship, often fathers teaching their sons. Their businesses were easily identified amid other shops – large carboys containing coloured water would often be placed in the shop window, sometimes with oil lamps or gas jets to illuminate them at night and cast an attractive multicoloured glow into the street. There was usually an outside lamp made of coloured glass. They packed their own remedies as well as selling nationally advertised patent medicines. To make their businesses viable, they sold other items that involved the use of chemicals or drugs: sauces, pickles

Walk 7

and spices, tea, cocoa, dyes, varnishes, ink, candles, lamp oil, wicks, matches and tobacco (which was not at that time seen as harmful to health). For the same reason, they were to be the main source of photographic products and services.

The transition from tradesmen to the profession of pharmacy took a step forward in 1841 with the establishment of the Pharmaceutical Society of Great Britain, based in Bloomsbury Square, in a building that had been flamboyantly remodelled in neo-classical style in 1778 by John Nash. To further the Society's educational aims, it founded a School of Pharmacy in the building. Lectures were offered in medical botany, chemistry, materia medica and pharmacy. From this evolved the basis of systematic training for pharmacy as a scientific profession with a sound academic base. This was given a boost in 1868 when the

Pharmacy Act enforced qualification by examination for those wishing to register as a chemist and druggist or as a pharmaceutical chemist. Various private schools also emerged to meet the growing need for formal, scientific training.

By 1918 the principle of a compulsory course of study was introduced in the UK. In 1925 the School became part of the University of London, and degree courses came to replace the traditional apprenticeship and private schools. The rapid development of pharmaceuticals in the 20th century required a similar growth in the number of pharmacists. The need to expand led the School of Pharmacy to move to a custom-built home in Brunswick Square in 1949, and in 1976 the Pharmaceutical Society also left Bloomsbury Square, moving to Lambeth. It acquired its 'Royal' designation in 1988.

of 'derangement'. At Fisher House, she had a room and a nurse/servant to herself, costing about £50–60 a year. Despite the widespread (and justified) view that many private madhouses were inhumane and a financial racket, Charles Lamb's descriptions support the view that some of them provided humane treatment. In 1811 the house was taken over by Alexander Sutherland, physician to St Luke's Hospital for Lunatics. It ceased to be a madhouse in 1836 and soon after was demolished.

Before moving on, Essex Road is noteworthy in the history of primary

care in London for one other reason. Following the introduction of smallpox inoculation in 1721, it was recognised that not only did the procedure endanger the recipient's life, but it also posed a threat to others. So 'airing houses', well away from the City, were needed to accommodate people until they had recovered and were no longer infectious. In 1746 what was to become the London Smallpox Hospital was established near Tottenham Court Road for this purpose, but this soon proved inadequate to meet demand. Two additional airing houses

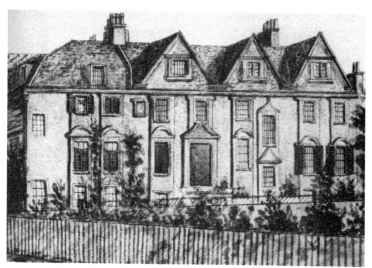

The rear of Fisher House, the private madhouse that in the early 19th century cared for Mary Lamb, 'the literary lunatic'. It was demolished in about 1840

were established, one of which was run by a Dr Poole in a house somewhere further out of town along Essex Road. Those with letters of recommendation would be called for their free inoculation, although they had to deposit £1 6d on admission to cover their funeral costs if they died – hardly reassuring. Although the house was quite remote, local residents were scared and opposed to the activity going on 'in their back yard' such that, to avoid abuse and insults, patients were advised to arrive and leave under cover of dark.

Walk back along Essex Road towards Islington Green and take the first right, Dagmar Terrace, at the top of which is the Little Angel Marionette Theatre, housed in what was built as the **Islington Temperance Hall**. Temperance halls were built all over the country in the second half of the 19th century to hold meetings to extol the virtues of abstinence and provide education and entertainment. This was in response to mounting concern about the damage that alcohol (p. 136), and gin in particular, was having on the health and well-being of the population. Two schools of thought emerged: those who felt that complete abstinence was the only way and those who advocated moderation. This has parallels with modern-day approaches to the management of heroin addiction.

Enter the gardens/graveyard of St Mary's Church through the gate to the left of the Temperance Hall. Walk past the front of the church to the first building on Upper Street, a fine red-brick building with its original use, **Islington Dispensary**, clearly indicated on the façade. As you can see, it was founded in 1821 and rebuilt in 1886 when it was necessary to widen the street

Walk 7

to accommodate the new public transport service, horse-drawn trams. You can see the patients' entrance and exit on the side of the building.

Unlike the one in Finsbury, Islington Dispensary depended not only on subscribers and donations, but also on small, regular contributions from those who might want to use the services if they became ill. Such 'provident' payments made up half the income in 1878 and were, in essence, a social insurance system. Payments were non-actuarial in that the amount did not depend on your likelihood of needing to use the services provided.

Islington Dispensary suffered minor bomb damage in 1940,

but rather than trying to struggle on after the start of the NHS, as Finsbury Dispensary did, it closed in 1946. However, as you have seen, the building continued to provide health care as the Islington Medical Mission used the building from 1949 until 1981. Following the Mission's closure, the building was converted to private apartments.

Walk back past the church along Upper Street, after 100 m turn left into Almeida Street, and at the end go through the alley to Milner Square. Turn right, walk through the square to Barnsbury Street, and then turn left towards Liverpool Road. The unusual turreted building on the opposite corner, together with the attached building in Barnsbury Street, was the **Islington**

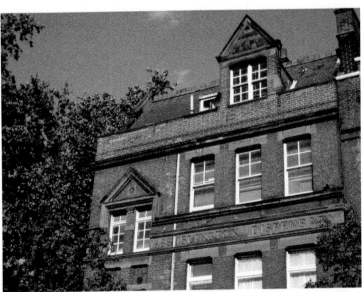

Islington Dispensary, a voluntary dispensary founded in 1821 to meet the needs of the fast-growing population, was rebuilt in 1886 to allow road widening for trams

Dispensaries

Until the middle of the 18th century, the only access to doctors for the poor and working class was in the outpatient clinics of the few hospitals. But from 1770 voluntary dispensaries were established that, in many ways, resembled present-day primary care (p. 211) centres. Compared with the outpatient departments, they were cheaper to provide and more geographically dispersed, and provided home visits for those too sick to travel. In addition, they provided an unrivalled opportunity for doctors to study diseases.

The first successful dispensary was established in Aldersgate Street. Several followed, such that by 1792 there were 16 in London. They followed a common plan, chiefly the design of one physician, John Coakley Lettsom. Many started in rented rooms or houses, but as the number of patients grew, some moved to larger, purpose-built premises. Like voluntary hospitals, they were established by concerned citizens (ideally including royalty and nobility). In return for an annual donation, subscribers were entitled to provide 'letters of recommendation' to members of the 'labouring and necessitous poor' to receive free care. Dinners, concerts and festivals were held to raise additional funds, and churches would dedicate a collection. In addition to providing medical treatment, dispensaries often had a Samaritan Fund to meet such social needs as food and clothing.

Dispensaries typically employed a resident apothecary and had several part-time physicians and surgeons; assistant posts were paid, others were honorary. The honorary staff were well established in their profession with private practices serving the middle and upper classes. The subscribers' influence extended to the choice of medical staff. As a result, candidates had to seek their support and votes. This reflected the importance to doctors of such posts. Assistant posts served as a stepping stone to posts at a major hospital.

The constant financial struggle that dispensaries faced led to two innovations in the mid-19th century. Many introduced a patient fee (or co-payment) not only to generate income, but also to reduce demand by discouraging 'misuse'. Patient payments soon accounted for as much as a quarter of a dispensary's income. More radical was the establishment of provident dispensaries, funded by working-class people contributing a small amount each week that entitled them to use the dispensary without charge when the need arose. Although a provident dispensary had been established in 1789, the movement really only got going in London in the 1830s. However, by 1870 there were still only 13, compared with 50 voluntary ones. By then, some Poor Law Unions had also established dispensaries for those so poor as to be entitled to outdoor relief.

Dispensaries gradually disappeared during the 20th century as alternative services emerged: National Health

Insurance introduced compulsory contributions for the low-paid, which meant that more people had access to those private doctors who participated ('the panel'); clinics devoted to particular needs (such as TB) were set up by charities and local government; and finally, from 1948, the NHS provided free primary care for all. Despite this, some voluntary dispensaries survived until as late as the 1960s.

Poor Law Relief Office & Dispensary.

In the 18th century, under the Elizabethan Poor Law, each parish had to provide 'necessary relief of the lame, impotent, old, blind and such other'. This was met in two ways: admission to a workhouse and the provision of 'outdoor relief'. The parish of St Mary's built its workhouse here in 1777. This initially accommodated 120 individuals but was extended so that, by 1814, it could house about 450. Islington was one of five parishes in London that was not assimilated into larger Poor Law Unions after the 1834 Act. The workhouse remained here until 1868 when the parish built a new one in Upper Holloway.

The original buildings were demolished and replaced in 1872 with those you see today. Built in what became known as Guardians' Gothic, they were for administering outdoor relief and for a Poor Law Dispensary, one of 47 established in England around this time. Staffed by a full-time dispenser and several part-time doctors (who were otherwise in private practice), it provided primary care for the poor and destitute of the parish. With the establishment of the welfare state

after World War II, the dispensary closed and the buildings were put to a number of uses before being converted in the 1990s for private homes.

Cross Liverpool Road and walk along Barnsbury Street (formerly Cut Throat Lane), past The Drapers' Arms to Thornhill Road. Turn left and walk past The Albion pub (one of the original 18th century tea gardens). Straight ahead, as you approach the next junction, you will see a handsome old shop front with Corinthian columns. Built around 1830, it is notable for the plate glass windows, which, at that time, represented the height of modernity. This was **Godfrey & Cooke's Dispensing and Family Chemist**, a private business that, like other pharmacists, made a modest but important contribution to providing primary health care. Behind each window would have been a large carboy containing coloured water with oil lamps or gas jets to illuminate them at night and cast an attractive multicoloured glow into the street. As with Wallis's pharmacy you saw earlier, there was also likely to be an outside lamp in coloured glass. In addition to dispensing medicines, pharmacists sold an eclectic collection of items,

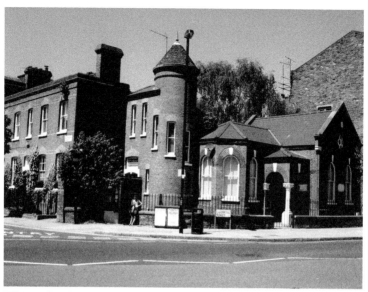

Islington Poor Law Relief Office (on the right), connected to the Poor Law Dispensary (on the left) by a circular stairway (in the turret), both being built in 'Guardians' Gothic' style in 1872

essentially anything related to treating and curing ill-health plus anything that involved chemicals, such as photographic equipment, turpentine, paraffin, perfumes and cosmetics, toiletries and cleaning agents. Perhaps relating back to their 'druggist' origins, chemists also sold tobacco, which was not at that time seen as harmful to health. A record of the range of items on sale can be seen in the extensive advertisements painted on the side wall, in Cloudesley Road.

Continue along Cloudesley Road and after 150 m turn left into Cloudesley Square. As you enter the square, note the small building (No. 18½) on the left, built in 1907 by Robert Stuart, who lived in the adjacent house. He had qualified

in medicine from Dublin in 1896 and, after practising from a house in Cloudesley Road for eight years, he moved here and added this purpose-built **GP surgery**. This was unusual – most GPs converted a couple of rooms in their own home. At that time, small social insurance 'clubs' run by Friendly Societies meant that increasing numbers were entitled not only to sickness benefit, but also to access to the 'club doctor', a GP who received an annual payment from the Society to provide all necessary care, including medications. GPs needed the income from being a club doctor but resented the club's interference in their work. Some clubs would instruct doctors how long they could spend with each patient,

Walk 7

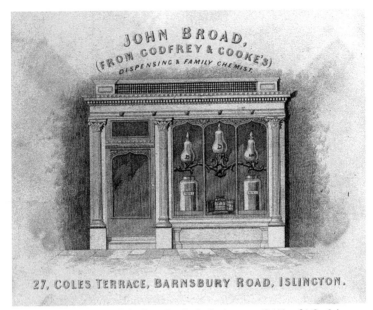

1830s' advertisement for John Broad, who had taken over Godfrey & Cooke's Dispensing & Family Chemist

banging on the surgery door when time was up!

By the start of the 20th century, government felt that insurance could not remain voluntary. In 1911 compulsory National Health Insurance was introduced for all employed workers with an income of less than £160 a year. They were required to pay four pence a week to an approved society, which was supplemented with three pence from their employers and two pence from the government. This entitled the insured worker (but not his or her family) to limited cash benefits when sick, the services of a GP and any prescribed pharmaceuticals (but not hospital treatment).

Instead of only the one club doctor, people could now choose their GP from all those on the 'panel' or list. In turn, GPs were free of the lay control exerted by the 'clubs' and remained independent contractors operating from their own premises. Robert Stuart left in 1915 (for Hertfordshire), and it is not known if the building continued to be used as a GP's surgery.

Walk past Trinity Church and leave the square on the far side onto Liverpool Road. Cross over. Turn right and stop after 30 m outside the entrance to Royal Free Place. Now a residential estate, this was the first infectious disease hospital (p. 78) in London, the **London Fever Hospital**. Despite local opposition from people fearful of the risks they would be exposed to (a view encouraged by some leading

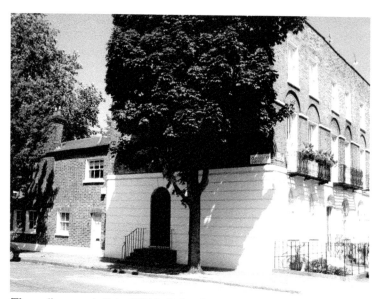

The small surgery, built in 1907 for Robert Stuart, a private general practitioner, onto the back of his house in Cloudesley Square

doctors including Thomas Wakley, editor of *The Lancet* and a local MP), the hospital, which replaced that at Battlebridge (King's Cross), was built. It opened in 1849 with 130 beds, although this was subsequently increased to 200. While the risk to local residents was, as supporters including Florence Nightingale had claimed, negligible, there were serious dangers for staff. Despite precautions, three of the first eight physicians and several nurses and other staff at the hospital died from the fevers they contracted.

The contribution of the hospital was appreciated by Charles Dickens, who became vice-president of the governors. In 1862 his view was that it was 'not only the single hospital of its kind in London but probably the best hospital of its kind in Europe'.

In common with the rest of the Fever Hospital Movement, the policy was not only to treat the patients, but also to whitewash the walls of their home, wash the clothes of the patients and their family members, and fumigate infected houses with nitrous acid solution. The hospital's links with the community extended to the provision of 'an appropriate vehicle' for the conveyance of patients to the hospital – possibly the first ambulances (p. 106) in London. The hospital was also appreciated by the more affluent, who wanted somewhere to confine their servants when the latter developed a fever and therefore threatened the health of their family. Some pay-beds were provided to meet this demand.

Walk 7

By the 1860s there was a growing realisation that London needed a coordinated service to respond to the danger and impact of infectious diseases. The Metropolitan Asylums Board (p. 179), established in 1867, created a comprehensive network of public fever hospitals across London, thus reducing the need for the London Fever Hospital. The need fell further as general hospitals became increasingly capable of coping with infectious diseases. The final demise of the Fever Hospital came during World War II when the building was requisitioned to handle trauma cases. It was allocated to the Royal Free Hospital to manage, an association that was made lasting in 1948 when the hospital became part of the Royal Free (hence its current name), mostly providing maternal and child services. It closed in 1974 when its 'parent' hospital moved from Gray's Inn Road to its new home in Hampstead.

Some of the original building, designed by Charles Fowler (architect of Covent Garden market), remains: the central building with a red-brick colonnaded façade in Palladian style (which housed the board room and administrative offices) and the two wings (containing the 'superior wards') connected by (recently reconstructed) archways. An Italianate fountain stood in the forecourt, with the wards crowded behind. If you go through the left archway, you can see, to your left and right, the only surviving ward blocks, with

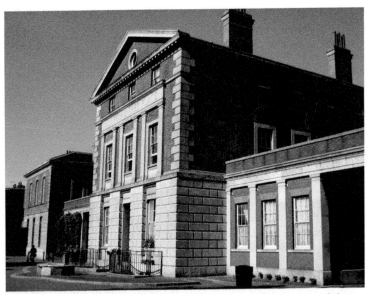

The central administrative block and one of the two lateral buildings containing the 'superior wards', which formed the grand frontage of the London Fever Hospital designed by Charles Fowler in 1849

first-floor balconies so that patients could benefit from the restorative properties of fresh air. The rest of the buildings are of recent origin.

Return to Liverpool Road, turn left and continue to the zebra crossing. Cross over and stop on the corner with Ritchie Street. The terraced houses about 30 m along on the left of Ritchie Street (after an arched vehicular entrance) disguise a purpose-built health centre for the **Ritchie Street Group Practice**. This is a modern primary care team of nurses, health visitors, doctors, midwives and counsellors.

It epitomises modern primary care in that a host of services in addition to medical consultations is provided, including family planning, minor surgery, immunisations, child development and diabetes clinics. In many ways, it has more in common with its 18th and 19th century predecessor, the dispensary, than it has with its more recent antecedent, single-handed private general practitioners of the early 20th century. This is the realisation of the Dawson Report's vision from 1920.

Also note No. 58, on the other side of Liverpool Road. From 1870

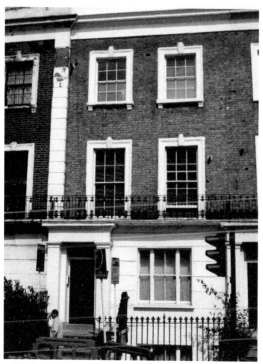

The Islington & North London Provident Dispensary occupied this house from 1870 to 1890, another example of how, until recently, primary care made use of domestic rather than specialised buildings

until about 1890, this was the home of the **Islington & North London Provident Dispensary**, geared to the needs of those who could and were prepared to insure for their future health care needs. The provident dispensary movement, which started in earnest in 1832, never took off in the way the earlier voluntary dispensaries had. By 1864, when this dispensary started, only 13 had been established in 32 years in London, and this one had only 678 members. It continued until 1890, by which time other means of funding and providing primary care were well established, developments that would lead to National Insurance and eventually the NHS.

Continue along Liverpool Road to Islington High Street where you can cross over to the Angel underground station, where the walk ends.

Motoring tour: No city is an island

Cities need their hinterland of towns and villages, and in turn towns and villages depend on cities. This relationship is as true for health care as it is for food, industry, education, defence and finance. Since the 18th century, London has provided health care not only for its own citizens, but also for those residing in the surrounding counties. In the late 19th century, 12% of the deaths in London hospitals were of patients from outside the metropolis. At the same time, London has depended on its rural neighbours to help meet some of the health care needs of its urban population. Like all symbiotic relationships, it was based on mutual advantage rather than exploitation.

Health care is an industry. Trade in patients brought financial benefits both to London and to the neighbouring areas. Nowhere was this truer than Dartford: during the first half of the 20th century, in and around the town, there were beds for about 8,000 patients from London. While the benefit to such towns was largely economic, London benefited in four ways: protection of its citizens (by exporting infectious patients); provision of more humane care (by sheltering the mentally ill and those with learning difficulties in rural asylums); freeing up of its acute hospital beds (by sending chronically ill patients to convalesce); and taking advantage of the 'healthier' rural and coastal environments.

With changes in health care policy, most of these activities ceased during the second half of the 20th century. However, many of the buildings that provided the services have survived. While these can be found throughout the home counties, north and east Kent has some of the finest examples of the interdependency that existed between London and its hinterland. There were asylums for the mentally ill (City of London Lunatic Asylum, Heath Asylum) and for those with learning difficulties (Darenth Schools). There were hospitals for those with infectious diseases (Southern Hospital). And there were convalescent homes for London hospitals (St Luke's Workhouse Infirmary, The London Hospital).

In addition, Kent offered something else unobtainable in the city – fresh air and sea-water. First proposed in the 17th century, the perceived health benefits of sea-bathing and sea air (particularly for treating tuberculosis) were widely accepted by the 19th century, leading to the establishment of hospitals (Royal Sea Bathing Hospital, Princess Mary's Hospital for Children) and later hydrotherapy institutions (Cliftonville Hydropathic). The perceived health benefits of the area attracted not only Londoners, but also people from further afield. In addition to private facilities for the affluent (including the aristocracy), many national organisations with working-class members established large convalescent homes (Railwaymen, Friendly Societies, Working Men's Clubs).

While the contribution of Kent in helping to meet the health care needs of Londoners is the key theme of this tour, there are three other themes. The first is the close relationship between civil and military health services. In the 18th and 19th century, both the army (Fort Pitt Hospital) and the navy (Royal Naval Hospitals at Chatham and Deal) established their own hospitals. And with Kent being the British front line in any European hostilities, the government and the military relied on the civil sector to provide additional facilities in times of conflict. During World War I, apart from depending on civilian hospitals, many establishments in Kent were converted to Auxiliary War Hospitals run by a vast unpaid workforce of nurses, the Voluntary Aid Detachments. Requisitions of civil buildings recurred in World War II.

Another theme is the development of the pharmaceutical industry. Before about 1900, drugs were largely naturally occurring compounds prepared and dispensed by apothecaries and pharmacists. Developments in chemistry led to the industrialisation and later the regulation of drug manufacture. Two of the key players in the development of the pharmaceutical industry in the UK were based in Kent: Silas Burroughs and Henry Wellcome established their main factory in Dartford in 1889 (and a materia medica farm alongside in 1904), and the US company Pfizer located its British (and later European) headquarters at Sandwich in the early 1950s.

'Health tourists' seeking benefit from sea-water in the 19th and early 20th century were not the first visitors to the area seeking salvation. While the sick and infirm had been drawn to Canterbury Cathedral since the 7th century, people flocked there after the murder of Thomas Becket in 1170. Belief in the healing properties of his shrine spread far and wide, attracting pilgrims not only from Britain, but also from abroad. Apart from the large infirmary that already existed beside the cathedral, hospitals were established in Canterbury (Eastbridge Hospital, St John's Hospital) and along the pilgrims' routes, such as at Sandwich.

While Kent has for centuries provided health services for outsiders – Londoners, sailors, the military, pilgrims – it has, like everywhere else, also had to meet the needs of its own people. In this, the pattern of services has been similar to that seen in other rural areas. There have been isolation hospitals, from medieval leper hospitals (St Bartholomew's Rochester, St Nicholas' Harbledon) to local smallpox hospitals (Whitstable). As in the large cities, there were workhouse infirmaries for the poor, voluntary dispensaries and hospitals, and asylums. Unlike cities, cottage hospitals (without resident doctors) were also developed from the 1870s onwards. They often commemorated individuals (David Livingstone in Dartford) or events (Queen Victoria's diamond jubilee at Herne Bay, the fallen of World War I at Whitstable). Although most have survived by adapting to changing needs, some have long since closed.

Kent Tour

While examples of all these themes recur throughout this tour, one or two themes tend to dominate each day. Much of the first day concerns the provision of hospitals to cope with London's need for care of its citizens with infectious diseases, mental illness and learning difficulties. In addition, meeting the needs of the army and navy also features. On the second day, the emphasis is on the perceived benefits of fresh air and sea-water to aid recovery and treat tuberculosis. And on the last day, the focus switches back to medieval times and the care of pilgrims. Meeting the needs of local people features throughout the tour.

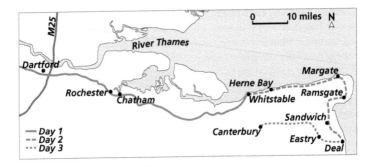

Day One: London to Whitstable

Highlights

- mid-19th century workhouse infirmary (Dartford Union Workhouse)
- two late-19th century lunatic asylums (Heath Asylum, City of London Asylum)
- largest number of hospital beds ever in one location in the UK (Darenth)
- oldest surviving hospital site in the UK (St Bartholomew's, Rochester)
- first military hospital for British army (Fort Pitt Hospital, Rochester)
- original home of the Army Medical School (Fort Pitt, Rochester)
- site of an early-19th century Naval Hospital (Melville Hospital, Chatham)
- the last Royal Naval Hospital to be built (Medway Hospital, Chatham)

The tour begins at the start of the A2 in Greenwich. Drive for about eight miles, leave the A2 at the Dartford Heath junction and take the A2018 towards Bexley. Go straight on at the first roundabout (towards Bexley) and left at the second roundabout into Pinewood Place. The two stone gateposts either side of the road mark the original entrance into **Heath Asylum**, named after its location here on Dartford Heath. Take the first left and park.

The asylum was one of seven built outside London by the London County Council in response to the 1890 Lunacy Act, which made local authorities responsible for providing care for those with mental illness (p. 66). By the time it opened in 1898, the enthusiasm for 'curing' patients had given way to a more pessimistic custodial outlook that sought to provide a refuge for patients and protection for the public. The 2,000 male and female patients were housed separately in 60-bedded wards, all of which were kept locked. It was renamed Bexley Asylum in 1905, despite local opposition that felt it would be 'a grave injustice to the district' and lower property values. A further change of name, to Bexley Hospital, occurred in 1930, reflecting changing attitudes towards mental illness. Some wards were unlocked, and patients started to be admitted on a voluntary rather than compulsory basis. The associated need for higher staffing levels was reflected in the construction of a nurses' home (p. 151), the fine three-storey building to your left, now called Pinehurst.

Following its incorporation into the NHS in 1948, the hospital continued to provide inpatient care for the people of south-east London until the 1960s, when a closure programme commenced, reflecting the new policy of 'care in the community' – trying to maintain people in their own homes. It finally closed in the 1990s and was demolished. Apart from the nurses' home and some mature trees, all that remains is the chapel (now a private health club), which you can

Kent Tour

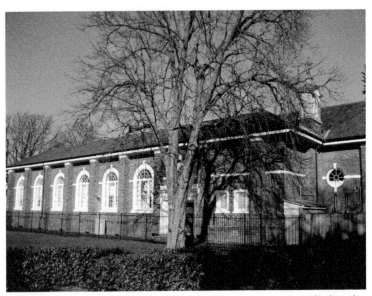

The Heath Asylum chapel (1899) could seat 850 men or women, but mixed services were not permitted. It now houses a private gym and health club

see ahead of you to the left. Built in 1899, the chapel could seat 850, although even here men and women were kept apart by holding separate services.

Return to the roundabout and follow the signs to Dartford (A2018). After 1.5 miles turn right at the T-junction onto West Hill. Descend the hill past a long yellow-brick building on your left, the former **Dartford Union Workhouse**, at the end of which turn left into Priory Hill and park.

Walk back towards West Hill and turn right into Twisleton Court, the 1836 workhouse for the newly formed Dartford Union (which covered 21 parishes). It replaced a 1729 building that served the local parish. The rear of the long entrance block on West Hill can be seen on

the left. The other buildings form a semi-circle, bisected by a central block that ends with a curved wall (painted white), which was the master's residence, affording him a view of all that took place. The rest of this block contained the kitchen and washhouse. The far side was for men (and included an accident ward), the near side was for women (including a lying-in ward).

Return to Priory Hill, turn right, and when you reach West Hill walk up the hill, past the original arched entrance to the workhouse, as far as a pathway on the right (Constance Grove). As the workhouse expanded up West Hill during the 19th century, it incorporated a police station, the small single-storey building with a pediment that can be seen further up West Hill.

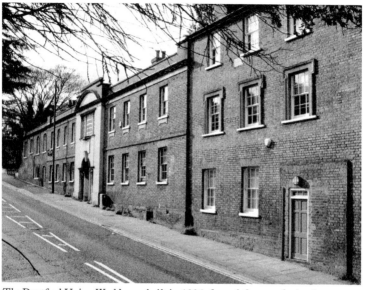

The Dartford Union Workhouse, built in 1836, formed the core of what became a large 19th century workhouse infirmary and, from 1948 until 2000, West Hill Hospital

Walk up Constance Grove. All that remains of the post-1836 buildings is the 1878 chapel to your right (awaiting redevelopment in 2012) and the wall that encircled the whole site, which, by the end of the 19th century, had become a large workhouse infirmary (p. 54). Following its transfer in 1930 to Kent County Council, it was renamed the County Hospital in an attempt to reduce any stigma attached to its origins. The name changed again in 1948, to West Hill Hospital, when it was incorporated into the NHS. It survived until 2000 when services were transferred to the new Darenth Valley Hospital. Walk past the chapel and return to Priory Hill through an opening in the wall ahead of you.

Drive on along Priory Hill, take the first right (Priory Place), and at the bottom turn right and immediately left onto Westgate Road (A220). Continue through several traffic lights and leave the town by the A226 (Greenhithe). Towards the top of East Hill, stop in the lay-by on the left opposite the **Livingstone Memorial Hospital**.

This cottage hospital (p. 271) was established in 1894 in memory of David Livingstone, the Christian missionary doctor and explorer who had died 21 years earlier. The hospital was opened by Henry Stanley (who had gone in search of Livingstone in Africa), whose speech kept the audience standing for over an hour. The more affluent locals were encouraged to subscribe by

Kent Tour

Silas Burroughs, one of the founders of Burroughs Wellcome, which had established its main factory in 1889 in the town centre beside the River Dart. The hospital consisted of two blocks connected by a covered way – an administrative block at the front (that you can see) and a ward block behind. The design of the front block is typical of cottage hospitals in its attempt to resemble a domestic dwelling. Among other services, it has provided maternity care, and in 1943 Mick Jagger and Keith Richard were born here.

Continue along the A226. About 500m after passing over the M25, a stone wall runs along the left side. This was the girdling wall for the **City of London Lunatic Asylum**. Turn left at the end of the wall (Cotton Lane) and then left into the old asylum site.

In 2012 it was being redeveloped for residential use, due for completion in 2014, so the extent of the site you can access will depend when you visit. This magnificent collection of buildings designed by James Bunstone Bunning opened in 1866 as an asylum for residents of the City of London. Despite its fine exterior with intricate stone-mullion windows and its fine grounds (including a cricket pitch), the interior was severely criticised in *The Lancet* as having 'cramped and draughty staircases, very defective toilets and was generally restricted by a spirit of parsimony'. Despite this, it was one of the first asylums to attract paying patients.

In 1887 it established its own farm (on the other side of Cotton Lane), primarily as a source of food for patients and staff rather than as

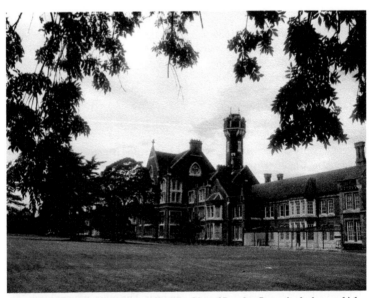

The majestic buildings and grounds of the City of London Lunatic Asylum, which opened in 1866. In 2012 it is being converted for residential use

occupational therapy for patients. The hospital was only partly successful as the depressed patients were largely inactive and those who were manic tended to abscond. The asylum became the City of London Mental Hospital in 1924, when voluntary patients were introduced, and Stone House Hospital in 1948, when it became an NHS hospital serving the local population rather than Londoners. Over the following 50 years, services were gradually reduced and it eventually closed.

Try to see the lawns and mature trees to the south of the main buildings and the 1901 flint chapel designed by Andrew Murray. It is unique not only in having two entrances (one for men, one for women), but also for the large porches to which epileptic patients seized by a fit during a service could be removed.

Turn right on leaving the hospital, then right onto the A226 (back towards Dartford) and first left (St Johns Road). At the crossroads after 500 m, turn right (Hillhouse Road), and after 50 m turn left onto the B2500. After 500 m, at a roundabout, turn right to Darenth. You are now driving along the western boundary of a site that was home to two massive health care institutions. It was over a mile from north to south and half a mile wide. After 500 m, turn left at the roundabout into Darenth Park Avenue. After 500 m, when the road turns to the left, park.

Take the path that runs diagonally away from the houses and stop at the gate into Darenth Country Park. You are at the heart of what was an immense complex

of public hospital buildings in the early 20th century. In 1903 there were beds for over 4,200 people on this site, a figure that has never been surpassed in the UK. The houses you have just driven past occupy the old site of the **Darenth Schools for Imbeciles**. Until 1867 people with learning difficulties (then referred to as imbeciles) were housed in workhouses. The newly created Metropolitan Asylums Board (p. 179) created two huge asylums, catering for all ages, to the north and to the south-west of London, but there was concern about incarcerating children with adults. There was a spirit of optimism that children could be improved and developed, a process that would be retarded by the presence of 'untrainable' adults. So, in 1878, this site was acquired and the Darenth Schools were built. A series of 13 ward blocks built along a corridor allowed free passage of air and light for the 580 children transferred here from London workhouses. The children were divided up: the healthy majority, the paralysed, infants, epileptics and the sick. The latter were housed in two infirmary blocks. There were schoolrooms, workshops for industrial training, kitchens, a laundry and a chapel.

It soon became apparent that the hope that many children could be trained and then returned to their homes was too optimistic. To avoid sending them to other adult asylums where any achievements might be negated, it was decided to build **Darenth Asylum for Imbeciles** alongside. It stood on

Kent Tour

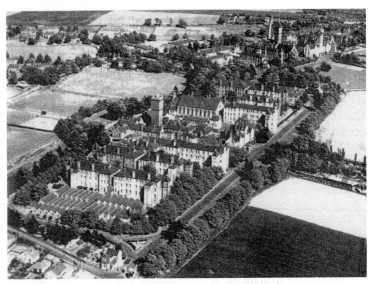

The vast complex of Darenth Schools for Imbeciles (1878) in the foreground, and beyond it Darenth Asylum for adults (1882)

the site occupied by the houses you can see on the higher ground from where you are standing. Although it was intended to accommodate 1,000 young adults with the capacity to benefit from training, some London workhouses took advantage of the opportunity to send elderly inmates. In 1882, a year after it opened, only 20 of the 220 patients were using the workshops. Soon, pressure on space led to the need for more adult accommodation, so in 1890 ten single-storey pavilions were constructed to the north of the asylum (beyond the houses).

By 1900, with over 2,000 patients, the emphasis shifted to teaching manual rather than intellectual skills. The workshops produced brooms, mattresses, books and metal goods to help provide

income and to pay patients a small salary. In 1935 the schools were closed as it was no longer deemed appropriate to institutionalise children, and the name changed to Darenth Park Hospital. Views were to change again, and in 1959 children were reintroduced. However, this new initiative was short-lived. By the 1970s the policy of 'care in the community' was established, leading to closure in 1988 and demolition in 1995.

Turn now to look at the fields and woods below you. This site was home to an enormous infectious diseases hospital (p. 78), the **Southern Hospital**. It was composed of two parts. If you look along the path ahead, there is a wooded area of high ground. This was the site of the Upper Hospital. The ground that falls away to the right was the site of the Lower Hospital.

In the 1880s the greatest threat to Londoners was smallpox epidemics. The Metropolitan Asylums Board (p. 179) created four new fever hospitals on the outskirts of London where victims could be isolated. The one at Deptford, which served south-east London, was overwhelmed during the 1881 epidemic, so a tented camp was established here beside Darenth Asylum (in the area between you and the new houses) for convalescent cases. This required the establishment of the first London-wide ambulance service (p. 106) for hospital patients, who were also transported by river ambulances along the Thames to Long Reach, north of Dartford, and then to here along specially laid granite roads.

A longer term solution was needed, so neighbouring Gore Farm (which lay down the hill below you) was acquired in 1883. During the 1884–85 epidemic, 10,000 cases were cared for in the 300 beds in the tents of Gore Farm Hospital. Between 1887 and 1890 the tents were replaced by 20 two-storey ward blocks on the high ground (the Upper Hospital), and in 1902 by ten single-storey ward blocks on the lower ground (the Lower Hospital). In 1908 the whole ensemble was renamed the Southern Hospital.

During World War I, the Upper was a US hospital for wounded servicemen, and the Lower became Dartford War Hospital for German POWs. Both parts reverted to an infectious diseases hospital after the war.

In World War II, it provided a safe home for the Royal Naval Hospital from Chatham. Following incorporation into the NHS in 1948, the Upper served as a general hospital and specialised in the care of polio victims until it closed in 1959. Part of the Lower was used from 1955 as Mabledon Hospital, a neurosis unit caring for Polish patients. In 1967 the Upper and much of the Lower were demolished to make way for the new A2 that cut across the site, leaving Mabledon Hospital on the far side until it too closed in 1985 and was demolished.

Walk down the path towards the site of the Southern Hospital. At the gate, bear right and after 20 m go into Southern Rest on the left, one of two cemeteries that served the hospitals. There are a few headstones dating from around 1900, the time of the last major smallpox epidemics. On leaving the cemetery, turn left, and in 20 m the path meets a wide track lined by horse chestnut trees. This was the main driveway leading to the Upper Hospital in the trees above you to the left. The Lower Hospital was to the right beyond the trees. Nothing remains of either site apart from a few forgotten bricks lying among the trees.

Return to your car and drive on. The houses you pass on your left were built on the site of the adult asylum. When you reach Darenth Park Avenue, turn right. This takes you to the only asylum buildings that remain – a house and the old Darenth Asylum Farm, now a riding school for disabled people. The asylum had not only a farm of 102 acres, but also a well and a gas-works (which closed in 1927 when electricity became available). To maintain segregation, only male patients were allowed to work on the farm.

Drive back along Darenth Park Avenue, passing **Darent Valley Hospital**, the new general hospital that opened in 2000 and replaced West Hill, Joyce Green and Gravesend & North Kent Hospitals. Turn right towards Bean, and after 1.5 miles join the A2. After six miles (when the M2 starts) stay on the A2 as it descends to Rochester and Chatham. After crossing the River Medway, continue along the A2, up Star Hill and along New Road towards Chatham. Shortly after passing **St Bartholomew's Hospital** on the left, turn right into Fort Pitt Hill and park.

The central block of St Bartholomew's, built in 1862 when the hospital was reconstituted as a voluntary general hospitals (p. 148), had blocks added at both ends later in the 19th century. In the 20th century, further ward blocks were constructed to the rear. The original appearance is much altered as a consequence of New Road being raised several metres, so that the hospital entrance had to be moved to the first floor, reached by a bridge from the pavement. In 1999 acute services were transferred, leaving it as a community hospital, although in 2012 its future is uncertain.

Although it would appear to be just another 19th century voluntary hospital of little historic significance, you are looking at the oldest surviving hospital site in the

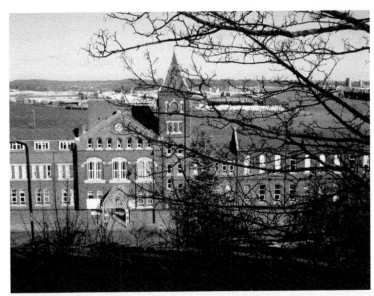

St Bartholomew's Hospital in Rochester overlooking the River Medway. The central block and tower (1862) were extended in the late 19th century

UK. Health care was first provided on this site in 1078, when Bishop Gundulph founded a hospital for leprosy (p. 17) outside the Rochester city wall. To see what remains of the original buildings, walk down to New Road, cross and go down Gundulph Road (to the right of the hospital) to Rochester High Street.

Before looking at the medieval remains of St Bartholomew's, cross the High Street to see the **John Hawkins' Hospital**. These 12 almshouses were established in 1592 for 'poor decayed mariners and shipwrights' by the explorer Sir John Hawkins (whose fortune partly came from establishing the slave trade between Guinea and the West Indies). They were rebuilt in 1790 for those with naval links. Hawkins, together with Francis Drake, was also responsible for establishing one of the earliest health insurance schemes in 1604, the Chatham Chest. Seamen who contributed weekly were entitled to support and pensions when they became disabled, infirm or aged.

Cross back to the flint and ragstone church, which, before the Reformation in the 1530s, was the St Bartholomew's Hospital chapel. It was restored by Giles Gilbert Scott in 1896 but in 2012 was in a sad state and awaiting redevelopment. This is all that remains of the medieval hospital that extended up towards New Road. The rear of the 19th and 20th century buildings can be seen, including a strange white 'castle', the origins and purpose of which are unknown.

Walk back up Gundulph Road, cross New Road and climb Fort Pitt Hill. After passing the University for Creative Arts building on the right, the road ends at gates into Fort Pitt Grammar School. The school occupies the site of Fort Pitt, one of three forts built in 1805–19 to protect the naval dockyards of Chatham from invasion from the south. However, by 1828, with the threat receding and the increasing numbers of injured soldiers returning to Chatham from overseas wars, a military hospital (p. 250) was needed. **Fort Pitt Hospital**, initially established in the existing barracks, was replaced in 1832 with an H-shaped, purpose-built hospital. Although a major improvement, the new hospital was inferior in design to the Melville Hospital, which had been built nearby for the navy six years earlier. The latter had 14 beds to a ward rather than 27 here.

Over the following 90 years, several additions were made, including an asylum to accommodate men 'labouring under insanity' (1847), facilities for soldiers' families (1860) and new ward blocks (1910). But the most significant development took place in 1860 with the establishment of the **Army Medical School**, which met a long-recognised need. It took the chaos and confusion experienced in the Crimean War plus a Royal Sanitary Commission report in 1858 and the enterprise and fortitude of Florence Nightingale to help set up the school. It was created in the stores building and provided a four-month course for 90 doctors a year in military medicine, covering the treatment of gun-shot wounds, tropical diseases, and military hygiene and sanitation. With the establishment in 1863 of a new military hospital at Netley near Southampton, the School moved there after only three years. It was later to move to even grander premises on Millbank in London.

The amount of the site you can see will depend on the time of your visit. If the school is open, you might obtain permission from the Headteacher's office to look around and see the remaining 'Crimea' wing of the 1832 hospital, a yellowish brick building to the left (east) of the site, and the red-brick ward blocks added in 1910. If you cannot gain access, you can still see two features of the hospital if you stand by the main reception entrance to the UCA building: directly ahead, you will see the end wall of the single-storey brick building that was the original home of the Army Medical School; and 30 m to your right is a fine two-storey brick building that was the hospital's asylum. Although Southampton replaced Chatham as

Military hospitals

Although magnificent Royal Hospitals were constructed for the army at Chelsea (1682) and for the navy at Greenwich (1694), their role was to accommodate retired and disabled servicemen rather than provide health care. Until the middle of the 18th century, the only hospital care for soldiers comprised small regimental facilities in their barracks, while sailors were treated in hospital ships moored in naval dockyards.

The first permanent Royal Naval Hospitals were Haslar Hospital in Portsmouth (1754) and Plymouth Hospital (1762). Others followed at Deal (1795), Great Yarmouth (1811), Chatham (1828) and Woolwich (1860). Meanwhile, although the army established several small hospitals between 1780 and 1820, the first major purpose-built facility was Fort Pitt Hospital at Chatham in 1832. With the port of arrival of wounded soldiers switching to Portsmouth, the

vast Netley Hospital was built. Despite its design attracting much criticism from the sanitarians, it opened in 1863, followed two years later by the Herbert Hospital in Woolwich. Others followed at Aldershot (1879), Colchester (1898) and again in Aldershot (1898). Finally, the Queen Alexandra Military Hospital on Millbank opened in 1905.

During the 20th century, military hospitals gradually closed in the face of declining needs in the UK, which could be met by civilian hospitals. However, both World Wars required temporary facilities to be created. During World War I all manner of buildings, particularly in Kent, were converted to Auxiliary War Hospitals staffed by Volunteer Aid Detachments. There were about 100 detachments, each comprising 20–50 staff (mostly women), which nursed over 125,000 injured servicemen.

the major port of entry for injured soldiers from the 1860s, the hospital did not close until 1922.

Return to your car, drive back down to New Road and turn right. After 0.7 miles, turn left at some traffic lights towards Chatham Town Centre. Follow the signs towards Chatham Maritime, and after about one mile you will see the main gate to the old Royal Dock Yard, where you should stop. On the opposite side of the road is a 1960s high-rise housing estate. This was built on the site of **Melville Hospital**, built for the navy six years before Fort Pitt Hospital. Before that, sick and injured sailors were cared for in hospital ships moored on the Medway or, from 1760, in the Marine Infirmary in the dockyard. The hospital, which faced the road, consisted of five buildings linked by a 90 m covered arcade. The central and end buildings were three-storey ward blocks, each containing six 14-bedded wards. Although it was replaced in 1905 by a new naval hospital about a mile away (which you will see in a few minutes), the buildings survived until the 1960s as Royal Marine barracks.

Drive on and turn right at the roundabout into Wood Street. Take the first right (High Street) and drive 100 m, past some shops, and stop in Brompton Hill. The 3 m high brick wall to your right marks the top of the Melville Hospital site. Opposite, under the grass mound behind railings, is a small reservoir to which water was pumped by the sawmill engine in the dockyard at night in order to supply the hospital.

Turn round and drive back along High Street and right onto Wood Street (which becomes Brompton Road). Follow the red H signs to the **Medway Maritime Hospital**. The route will take you along Rock Avenue and then, at some traffic lights, right along Montgomery Road, at the end of which is the hospital. Before reaching the hospital, turn into a side street and park. You can explore the hospital site on foot. On entering, turn left along the perimeter road and stop.

The perimeter wall and the impressive gatehouses at the entrance are evidence of its origins in 1905 as the Royal Naval Hospital that replaced the Melville Hospital. The original building is hard to discern after 100 years of modifications and additions. It is hard to make out the shape and style of the original, although some parts are visible. The Italianate clock tower still dominates the site, and you can glimpse parts of the ward blocks – red-brick pavilions with stone bands, domes and huge decorative arches, reminiscent of Westminster Cathedral. You will get a better view in a few minutes. The other interesting feature is the series of buildings constructed as staff residences round the outer edge of the site. Many have been converted for clinical use, but some of their former roles can be seen, such as the Surgeon Rear Admiral's residence (No. 8).

Walk on round the site to the back of the main buildings where you can see a massive water tower and two of the original ward blocks, which seem large, heavy and forbidding. Two great sanitary towers

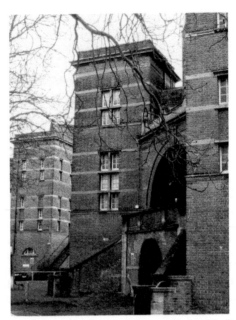

The imposing sanitary towers at the rear of the ward blocks of the Royal Naval Hospital, built in Chatham in 1905 and now part of the Medway Maritime Hospital in the NHS

stand guard beside huge arched entrances, which seem to have been built for giants rather than humans. And beneath the elevated first-floor entrances, a dark arched entrance suggests a cave or grotto rather than a welcoming, caring environment. Altogether an unusual style for a hospital of any era, which maybe reflects the fact that the original clientele were members of the armed services rather than civilians. With the demise of Chatham as a major naval base after World War II, the hospital closed in 1961, reopening in 1965 as Medway Hospital (part of the NHS), and in 1999 it was renamed Medway Maritime Hospital to reflect its naval heritage.

Return to your car, drive back to Rock Avenue and turn right. At the T-junction turn left onto the A2 (towards Sittingbourne). At the roundabout after 1.6 miles, turn right towards the M2 and then, after 2.2 miles, left onto the M2 (Dover). After 16 miles the M2 ends and you should take the A299 towards Margate. Drive for 4.5 miles before exiting onto the A2990 (Whitstable). At the second roundabout, turn right onto the A290 towards Canterbury. After half a mile, turn left into Bogshole Lane. Stop by Seeshill Farm, a small white farmhouse on the left after 0.8 miles.

The dilapidated, ivy-clad flintstone barn at the roadside is still known locally as the **hospital for incurables**. Following the smallpox epidemic of 1884, this was established as an isolation facility for victims from Whitstable, a couple of miles away. Two old ship's cabins (long since disappeared) were used as a kitchen and a washhouse, and two earth closets were built. During epidemics, the erection of three hospital tents meant that 11 patients could be accommodated. As often happened, a beerhouse was opened (in what is now the farmhouse) to provide some comfort for the sick and refreshment for those who cared for them. Despite there being no further smallpox epidemics after 1904, the beerhouse continued as a pub until the 1920s.

Drive on and at the T-junction turn right (A2990). At the roundabout, turn left (signposted 'Cemetery') along Millstrood Road. At the bottom it curves to the left (Belmont Road) and ends at traffic lights by a railway bridge. Turn right along the High Street into the centre of Whitstable, where the first day of this tour ends.

Kent Tour

Day Two: Whitstable to Deal

Highlights

- convalescent homes for two London hospitals (The London Hospital, St Luke's Workhouse Infirmary)
- three World War I auxiliary war hospitals (in Tankerton and Herne Bay)
- three cottage hospitals (Whitstable & Tankerton, Herne Bay, Margate)
- two convalescent homes for national organisations (Herne Bay, Pegwell)
- finest Georgian sea-bathing hospital in UK (Royal Sea Bathing Hospital, Margate)
- seaside hospital for London children with TB (Princess Mary's Hospital, Margate)
- 1920s' hydro for water and electrical therapies (Cliftonville Hydro)
- 19th century voluntary dispensary (Ramsgate)
- 13th century hospital for foreign pilgrims to Canterbury (Sandwich)

Leave Whitstable, passing the harbour, and after about 400 m bear left up Tower Hill. Just before the brow of the hill, you will pass No. 6 Marine Parade, on the right. Like so many domestic properties in Kent, this served as a nursing home during World War I for servicemen who had been exposed to gas attacks in the trenches. After another 400 m stop by The Marine Hotel, with its impressive Dutch gable dormer windows.

When the four houses that the hotel occupies were built in 1899, they stood in splendid isolation on an unmetalled road on this cliff top site. No. 1, on the far right, was originally the **London Hospital Convalescent Home**. Like other London hospitals, it needed to ship its chronically ill patients out of the city, partly to vacate beds for acutely ill patients and partly because it was believed that fresh sea air would aid patients' recovery. Then, during World War I, the home, together with the three adjoining houses, was commandeered for **Tankerton Military Hospital**, which accommodated 300 injured servicemen. After the war, Nos 1 and 2 served as a civilian hospital until 1921, when the four houses were converted into The Marine Hotel. The hotel bar is located in what was Ward G.

Drive on along Marine Parade and take the second right (Pier Avenue) and then the second left (Northwood Road), where you will see the **Whitstable & Tankerton Cottage & Convalescent Hospital**. Like many cottage hospitals, it was established as a memorial to 'our fallen heroes' of World War I. It opened in 1926 (as recorded in Art Deco metalwork on the balcony above the entrance) and originally provided care not only for locals, but also for convalescent patients from London. It now is confined to meeting local needs.

Continue, turn left (Ellis Road) and then right onto Tankerton Road. Take the first exit at the mini-roundabout after 0.7 miles (B2205). In one mile

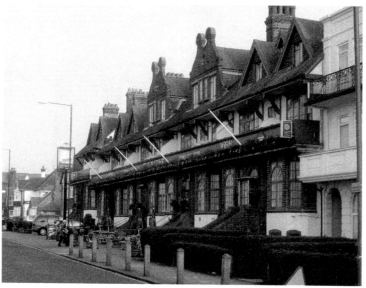

During World War I, these houses were requisitioned for Tankerton Military Hospital, staffed by a Voluntary Aid Detachment. The right-hand house had previously served as a convalescent home for the London Hospital in Whitechapel

you will pass the 'Herne Bay' sign. After a further 0.4 miles, turn left along Hampton Pier Avenue. At the pier, continue to the right along the sea shore (Western Esplanade). **Sea-water baths** were established in Herne Bay in 1792, and by 1883 the Registrar General for England declared it to be 'the healthiest watering place' in the country. As you approach the pier, note the 12-storey block of flats opposite. These replaced the 19th century Pier Hotel, which in 1898 became one of two convalescent homes for children from London workhouses established by the Metropolitan Asylums Board. You will see the other one in Margate later on.

Just after the clock tower, turn right (Market Street), and at the end turn left and then first right into William Street. Turn first left into High Street and then immediately left (New Street). Stop after 50 m, opposite the headquarters of the Herne Bay Division of **St John Ambulance**. The Order of St John is heir to the Hospitallers, the medieval religious order of knights formed in 1099 at the time of the crusades, which was committed both to nursing and to 'fighting the infidel'. In 1877 the Order created the St John Ambulance Association, dedicated to training volunteers in first aid and nursing. From 1879 volunteers formed themselves into ambulance and nursing corps, the first in the UK being in Kent. By 1887 there were so many corps that the Order united them as the

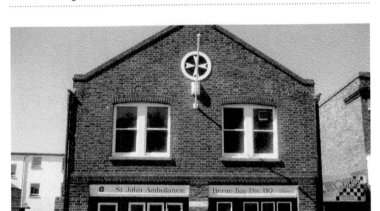

The St John Ambulance Station has used this old stable block in Herne Bay since 1930

St John Ambulance Brigade. By 1912 there were 25,000 volunteers. The Association (responsible for training and supplies) and the Brigade were eventually brought together as St John Ambulance.

This fine former stable block has been the headquarters of one of the 3,000 divisions in the UK since 1930. With 60,000 volunteers, the organisation treats 200,000 casualties a year. The organisation's symbol, the Maltese cross, which you can see on the building's façade, is a reminder of a key chapter in the history of the Order when, having been expelled from Rhodes in 1523, the Hospitallers found sanctuary in Malta for 275 years.

This short street has another connection with health care. The original home, from 1892 to 1901,

of **Herne Bay Cottage Hospital** was the three-storey white house opposite the St John Ambulance headquarters. You will visit its present location in a short while.

Continue along New Street as it turns to the left and then take the first left, South Road, which takes you back to the High Street. Turn right and then third left into Canterbury Road. Turn right into Beacon Hill and stop after 20 m, opposite Nos 5 and 6. These two interconnected houses were where many local people were born during the first half of the 20th century. With fine sea views, this was **St Brelade's Maternity Home**. Although lying-in hospitals had been established by surgeons in large cities from the mid-18th century, most childbirth (p. 22) continued to be managed by midwives outside hospitals until the 1950s. With poor housing conditions widespread, religious and other philanthropic organisations established homes where poor women could give birth in reasonable conditions, attended by a midwife. The involvement of doctors was minimal. From the 1950s onwards, home births gradually disappeared and the thousands of maternity homes were replaced by obstetric departments in general hospitals and, to a lesser extent, by maternity beds in cottage hospitals. Reflecting demographic changes, this building is now a nursing home for elderly people.

Drive on, take the first right (Beacon Road), then the first left (Beltinge Road) and then the first right (Downs Park). Stop opposite the first house on the right, No. 1. This was yet another residential property used as an auxiliary war hospital during World War I. A **Voluntary Aid Detachment** nursed 27 beds for injured soldiers from the Expeditionary Force here. Carry on along Downs Park. At the end, turn left into Mickleburgh Hill, at the top of which turn left into King Edward Avenue. Stop outside the **Queen Victoria Memorial Cottage Hospital**.

This, the third and present home of the cottage hospital, was custom-built in 1936. Compared with the architectural embellishments of 19th century hospitals, it is rather austere and featureless. It lacks both the domesticity of many cottage hospitals and the civic pride that most voluntary hospitals display. Various additions have been made over the years, the most interesting of which are some wooden huts behind the original building, which can be seen from the main car park on the right. These were probably erected as a temporary measure during World War II but are still in use 70 years later.

Continue along King Edward Avenue (which becomes Grange Road) to a T-junction. The houses on your left were built on the site of a fine mock-Elizabethan house that from 1902 to 1934 housed the **White Lodge Private Hydro**. Established and run by Dr Percival Vivian, it was 'intended to meet a need often felt by medical men, for a suitable place to send convalescent patients of the middle and wealthier class'. London doctors would send their patients for therapies based on water and electricity.

Turn right into Reculver Road and stop after 100 m outside Elliot House, on the left. Built in 1901, this was the first **Railwaymen's Convalescent Home**. It was established by a group of concerned railway managers and staff. The original home, designed by Sexton Snell, accommodated 100, such that in 1903, 725 railwaymen benefited from at least two weeks' free convalescence. Demand could not be met, so it was extended over the following 30 years to accommodate 265. In addition, in 1911, a second home opened on the Wirral, and eight more followed over the following 40 years. They relied on railwaymen's weekly subscriptions boosted by donations from the private railway companies. This home functioned

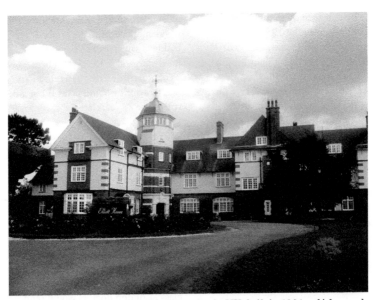

The first convalescent home for railwaymen in the UK, built in 1901, which served as an auxiliary military hospital in both World Wars

until 1979 and has since reopened as a private nursing home for 70 elderly people.

Fifty metres further along, you will see the magnificent green ornate gates of its erstwhile neighbour, the **Friendly Societies Convalescent Home**. Built two years before its neighbour, it was paid for by John Passmore Edwards, a philanthropist who had made his fortune in newspaper publishing. Often dubbed 'the English Andrew Carnegie', he funded public libraries, hospitals and convalescent homes all over the country. The two convalescent homes (p. 92) here served as a 225-bedded Auxiliary War Hospital during both World Wars. It was demolished in 1985, and only the gates survive.

Continue to the end of Reculver Road, turn left, and at the roundabout take the A299 towards Margate. At the roundabout after five miles, take the A28 (Margate). After 3.5 miles you will enter Margate, and at the first traffic lights turn left into St Mildred's Road (signposted to Westgate railway station). Immediately after crossing the railway line, turn right (Station Road), then third left into Adrian Square and stop.

The first large detached house on the left (No. 21), with a square, four-storey tower, served as a convalescent home for children from St Luke's Workhouse Infirmary in Chelsea but only for two years, from 1901 until 1903. It could accommodate 31 children for whom it was felt fresh sea air would aid their recovery from tuberculosis (p. 218). Its short existence may have resulted from it not being welcomed by the private prep schools that shared the square.

Drive on through the square, turn right onto Westgate Bay Avenue, and after 500 m take the fifth turning on the left, Royal Esplanade, along the sea front. At the end, the road turns right (Westbrook Gardens), where you should park. Walk back to the Royal Esplanade, where you can see one of the most spectacular locations for a hospital in Britain, the old **Royal Sea Bathing Hospital**, subject to redevelopment since 2005. The restored red-brick ward block was built in the 1880s. Behind it, the pediment and clock on the front of

Water

From medieval times, spring water was seen as having therapeutic properties. By the 17th century, doctors would refer patients to the dozens of spas being constructed around such sources. While people purportedly visited for the medicinal waters, spas became the fashionable place to be and to be seen.

By the 18th century, belief in the therapeutic benefits of water had extended to bathing, particular in sea-water. While this led to the development of numerous establishments along the south and east coasts for Londoners, sea-water baths were also created in London.

Meanwhile, the importance of clean water was well recognised after John Snow demonstrated the link between polluted water and cholera in 1854. The lack of clean drinking water, which contributed to the high levels of consumption of alcohol (p. 136), gave rise to the temperance movement and to the Metropolitan Free Drinking Fountain Association. From 1859 the latter erected many public fountains throughout London. By 1888 Charles Dickens estimated that 300,000 people drank from the 800 fountains each

day, along with 1,800 horses, creating a gathering place for people.

With no adequate water supply in many homes until the 20th century, washing was difficult. From 1846 local authorities were encouraged to build public baths and washhouses, including swimming baths and slipper baths (so-called because of the Victorian sense of modesty in draping bath-towels over the bath to conceal their bodies and in doing so making the bath look like a huge slipper). Baths were seen as improvers not only of health, but also of morals.

By the 1860s there was increasing interest among doctors in the health benefits of more specialised baths, imported from Turkey, so much so that they were installed in some hospitals. In addition, over 100 Turkish baths were set up as private establishments in London, most during the late 19th century.

A more controversial therapy was the use of cold water shock, a treatment that had been strongly espoused by John Wesley, who, like many clerics in the 18th century, studied and practised medicine as a hobby. On one occasion, he himself plunged into the Thames to stop a violent nosebleed. Belief in cold water shock was shared by some doctors, such as a Dr Doucet, who, in the 1820s, failed to convince his colleagues at the Royal Society of Medicine that throwing 15–26 buckets of cold water over tetanus patients would cure them. However, one area where it was used routinely until the mid-19th century was cold water plunges to shock lunatics out of their insanity.

Belief in the therapeutic power of water extended into the 20th century. In 1904 a Monsieur Quinton extolled the benefits of subcutaneous injections of diluted sea-water, which had to be collected from several miles out and from a depth of 10 m. For several decades, he successfully maintained two Sea-Water Dispensaries in London that provided 'Plasma of Quinton'.

the original 18th century building can just be seen.

The health benefits of water (p. 259) and, in particular, sea-bathing had first been promoted in the 1660s and became fashionable when it was claimed to have cured George III in the late 18th century. The General Sea Bathing Hospital was established here by the London physician John Coakley Lettsom in 1791 for those with chronic bone diseases (most notably TB). Margate could be reached easily from London by hoy (boat). The hospital had 30 beds in four wards, each having open colonnaded piazzas so that patients could be nursed out of doors.

Descend and walk along the promenade past the hospital. You can see the cobbled ramps that in summer allowed horse-drawn bathing machines to take patients to the beach so they could be fully immersed in the sea. The fine three-storey yellow brick building with the name proudly emblazoned facing the sea was added (at right angles) to the original 1791 building in the 1820s. A smaller building (which you will see in a few minutes) was added to the inland end, thus creating an H-shaped hospital.

After passing the hospital, take the steps back up, turn right and walk along Westbrook Road to Canterbury Road. The nurses' home on the corner was awaiting conversion in 2012. Walk along to the main entrance to see the wing added in 1820 to create the H-shaped hospital. It has a monumental Doric portico (salvaged from a villa), echoed by matching Doric pilasters decorating the wings on either side. In the 1830s single-storey pavilions were added at both sides.

The portico has not, however, always been here on the south side of the hospital. From the 1820s until the 1880s, it was on the west-facing (left-hand) side of the original 1791 building, which lies behind the building you can see. The person responsible for moving it was Erasmus Wilson, whose statue occupies pride of place in front of you. He was a highly successful London doctor specialising in skin conditions who encouraged daily

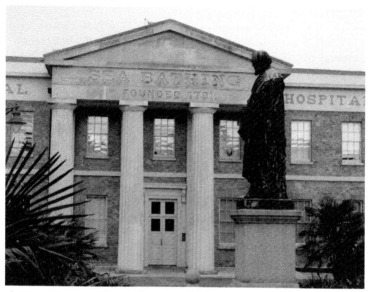

A statue of Erasmus Wilson in front of the fine Doric entrance to the Royal Sea Bathing Hospital, Margate

baths and introduced Turkish baths as therapy. Despite a profitable private practice, he was committed to alleviating the sufferings of the poor. Funding the hospital expansion here was only one of his philanthropic acts.

Unusually, Wilson does not face and greet visitors but instead looks to the west at the red-brick ward blocks surmounted by a yellow stone balustrade that he funded. Their addition meant that the west-facing entrance to the hospital became enclosed, so the entrance had to be moved to where you see it today. The flat roof of the ward blocks provided an area for patients to promenade. With the addition of an indoor salt-water bath, pumped up 30 feet from the sea, the hospital was able to stay open throughout the year.

As tuberculosis declined during the 20th century and effective drug therapies were introduced, the hospital was increasingly used for convalescence. It eventually closed in 1996, although its memory is preserved in a Sea Bathing Unit in the local hospital that looks after patients with arthritis. Carry on along Canterbury Road and turn right along Westbrook Gardens to return to your car.

Drive on along Westbrook Gardens, left into Canterbury Road and straight on into Margate along Marine Drive (beside the beach). At the mini-roundabout, go straight over (to the right of the clock tower) along Queen Street. Continue though Cecil Square and then straight on along Union Crescent and Addington Road. At the

Kent Tour

T-junction turn left and immediately right into Thanet Road, and park.

Walk back to see the building on the right-hand corner, a typical example of cottage hospital architecture. In 1876 **Margate Cottage Hospital** was established here in the single-storey cottage by the junction. With the addition of the three-storey building alongside it in 1897, it could accommodate 21 patients. This was increased to 31 in 1913 with the extension along Addington Road. In 1930 the hospital moved to a site outside the town, which you will see soon, since when this building has had many uses, including as a public library.

Continue along Thanet Road and left into Park Road, and at the crossroads go straight into Wilderness Hill. Park near the top and walk on up to Northdown Road at the top. During the 19th century, many institutions were established in this area for poor children from London who it was felt would benefit from sea air and sunshine. A few hundred metres to the left, the Metropolitan Infirmary for Children was established in 1841 for workhouse inmates with TB. In 1900 it became the West Ham Children's Convalescent Home, surviving until 1935, when it was demolished.

Immediately on your left, East Cliff House (in 2012 the local headquarters of Mencap) was acquired in 1895 by the St Pancras Poor Law Union as a convalescent home for 41 workhouse children. Two

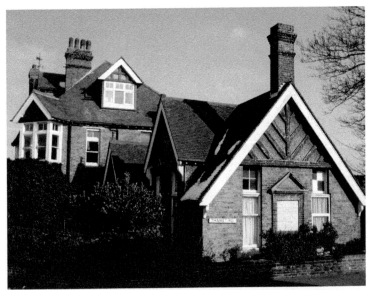

Margate Cottage Hospital, established in the single-storey cottage in 1876, with the three-storey building added in 1897. It moved to larger premises in 1930

years later, when the Metropolitan Asylums Board took over responsibility for Poor Law children throughout London, they made this home and St Anne's in Herne Bay (the site of which you saw) their two main facilities. Over the next 84 years, the home extended down the hill behind East Cliff House. It was designated **Princess Mary's Hospital for Children** in 1918.

Walk back down Wilderness Hill, and turn into the car park on the right between two white pebble-dashed buildings. The building to the right, with four gable ends protruding, was the first to be added (1901) and provided accommodation for 50 children mostly suffering from non-pulmonary TB (mostly disease of the bone). Two years later, a veranda was added along the length of the

building so children could be nursed in the open air. In 1930 responsibility for the hospital passed to the London County Council, which in 1934 converted it to Princess Mary's Convalescent Hospital for Women, reflecting the declining prevalence of childhood TB. Apart from closing temporarily during World War II, the hospital continued until 1981. The buildings are now residences and a nursing home.

Return to your car and drive up to Northdown Road, turn right, and then take the second on the right (Cliftonville Avenue) and park. In 1926 tourism here was at its height, and a nearby hotel acquired No. 6 as an annex. (The embedded 'A1' and '1902' refer to the year the first British submarine, the A1, was built.) Recognising the fashion

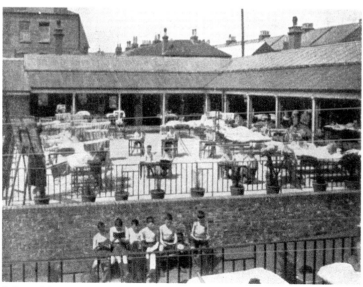

Princess Mary's Hospital for Children was established in 1895 to provide fresh sea air and sunshine for children with TB from London workhouses

for therapies based on water and electricity (p. 69), the proprietors added **Cliftonville Hydro**, the two-storey, white glazed building alongside. An additional storey was added later for staff accommodation.

The Hydro contained Turkish, Russian and electric baths. Only the wealthy could afford the services offered, which included a Vichy douche (massage under sprays of warm water), a bath in which you were invigorated by a mild electric current, ultraviolet sunlamps and the Bergonie Chair for treating obesity through rhythmical muscle contractions. By 1932 financial difficulties led to the Hydro being sold to the town corporation, which subsidised its use by local people until its closure in World War II. Since the 1960s, when the ground floor frontage was altered, it has been used as offices. Peer through the doors to see signs of its original use: the entrance hall is lined with marble, and the mosaic floor has a crescent and star motif, as do the stained glass windows to the left of the entrance.

Drive on down Cliftonville Avenue, turn right and after 30 m turn left onto Dane Road. Take the first right (Addiscombe Road), continue to the second mini-roundabout, and follow the signs to Broadstairs (A255). After 200 m, turn right into the Queen Elizabeth the Queen Mother Hospital (QEQM) site and then immediately right to park in front of **Margate & District General Hospital**.

Compared with the domestic architecture of its predecessor (the cottage hospital on Victoria Road), this 1930 replacement has echoes of a grand chateau. This reflects its transition to a general hospital. The central block, with an entrance surmounted by a copper tower, and two wings forming an H-shaped building can be seen. There were 80 beds and an operating theatre. The original name can be seen over the entrance, together with a stone bas-relief of a fruit tree entwined with two snakes (a confusing mixture of Eden, local orchards and Aesclepius, the god of healing). The confusion continues in the bas-relief above in that the hospital is named MH (Margate Hospital). In 1948 it became part of the NHS, since when it has expanded into a large general hospital serving the whole of Thanet. It now forms part of the Queen Elizabeth the Queen Mother Hospital.

Turn right out of the car park back onto the A255. Pass the 18th century Dutch-style almshouses on the right, and after 1.9 miles turn right (just after a school) into Fairfield Road. After 1.3 miles turn left onto the A254 to Ramsgate. After one mile cross the A255 into Chatham Street, and in 200 m bear left onto the High Street. Take the first left into Church Hill and park by the church where the road turns right into Broad Street. You will see, on the right, the old **Ramsgate & St Lawrence Dispensary**. Established elsewhere in 1820, it was officially known as the Royal Dispensary following a royal visit in 1824. It moved to these purpose-built premises in 1878, but, mysteriously, permission to use the 'Royal' prefix was withdrawn by the government in 1901. Like many other voluntary dispensaries (p. 229), it closed in 1948 with the introduction of free care from NHS general practitioners. Although it has been converted for residential use, its origins have been preserved in the fine lettering over the main entrance.

Drive back down Church Hill to High Street, turn left and then second right (George Street). Take the second on the left (Effingham Street), and at the T-junction turn right into Queen Street (which becomes West Cliff Road). After 300 m park near the old **Ramsgate General Hospital**. First, look at the large detached Georgian house opposite, home to a nursery school in 2012. It was built in 1849 as the **Ramsgate Seamen's Infirmary**, paid for by townsfolk concerned about the lack of hospital care for injured and sick sailors and fishermen. It had 20 beds and a resident nurse. Despite its purpose, members of the public were also admitted when there were spare beds. Increasing use by the public was reflected in name changes, first in 1891 to the Ramsgate Seamen's Infirmary & General Hospital and then in 1898 to the Ramsgate General Hospital & Seamen's Infirmary.

Increasing demand led in 1909 to the construction of the elegant two-storey building with dormer windows on the other side of the road. The hospital gradually expanded with additions during the 1920s of a children's

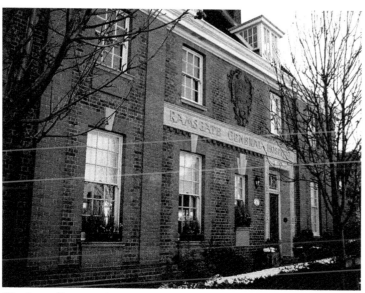

The elegant Ramsgate General Hospital (1909), which expanded throughout the 20th century but eventually closed in 1998 and has been converted for housing

Kent Tour

ward, nurses' home and maternity ward. To the right of the original building, a casualty and outpatients department was constructed in 1948 as a memorial to those who died in World War II. The front wall, including the commemoration stone, have been preserved. The hospital was incorporated into the NHS in 1948 and survived until 1998 when services were transferred to the QEQM Hospital.

Drive on along West Cliff Road, go straight on at the roundabout, and after 400 m bear left along Pegwell Road. After another 400 m turn into Pegwell Bay Hotel car park on the right. From the other side of the road, you can look down to see how the hotel extends down the cliff. In 1893 the philanthropist Passmore

Edwards purchased the hotel as a convalescent home for the **Working Men's Club & Institute Union**, a nationwide organisation with 460 clubs and 90,000 members. He had the building restored, together with extensive beachside gardens with gazebos. In 1898 the home was extended by the construction, on the other side of the road, of a new wing with a magnificent viewing tower. Men stayed about three weeks, enjoying the sea air, gardens and maybe even some shrimping – Pegwell was also known as Shrimpville – thanks to the plentiful supply of shrimps in the bay. In 1969 severe flood damage to the ground floor of the original building proved too expensive to repair and the convalescent home closed. It is

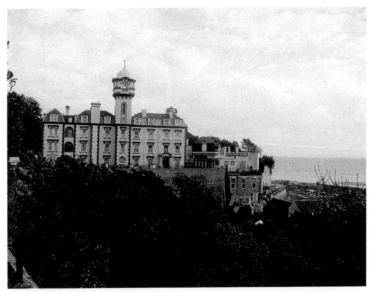

A convalescent home for the Working Men's Club & Institute Union was established in the hotel on the cliff face in 1893. The imposing addition in 1898 included an observation tower

now once again a hotel, although the gardens remain abandoned.

On leaving the hotel car park, turn right and continue along Pegwell Road. At the first roundabout turn left, at the second go straight on, and at the third take the first exit (A256) to Little Cliffsend Farm. After 3.4 miles there is a small roundabout. Take the first exit along the coast towards Great Stonar, which passes through what was built to house **Pfizer's European Headquarters**. Whereas Burroughs Wellcome was founded in England by two Americans, Pfizer was founded in the USA by two Germans. Charles Pfizer and Charles Erhart established the company in Brooklyn in 1849. It was to be 100 years before the company's commercial breakthrough in 1949 when the antibiotic oxytetracycline was discovered and marketed. In 1952 the company established a factory at Folkestone to process bulk imports of the drug. However, the government limited the quantity they could import in order to encourage Pfizer to manufacture in Britain. At the time, this area, known as Sandwich Haven, consisted of low-lying, roofless buildings, overgrown rail track and rusting dock installations. Fifty years later, after Pfizer had merged with several other drug companies, this 340-acre site had become their European headquarters for research and development, employing 3,600 people. The 21st century urban architecture is somewhat surreal among the medieval villages and 19th century seaside resorts of

east Kent. And in 2012, with the announcement of the end of their operations here, the future of the site is uncertain.

Continue on into Sandwich. Cross the River Stour and go straight on (round the medieval gateway) along the High Street. At the end, turn left into New Street. After 200 m you cross a railway line, and after a further 150 m park by the entrance to **St Bartholomew's Hospital**. Walk up the lane to the church and the encircling almshouses.

A medieval hospital (p. 35) to accommodate travellers from mainland Europe visiting Thomas Becket's shrine in Canterbury Cathedral was established here in 1190 (20 years after Becket's murder). Given that Becket's shrine was believed to restore health, many of the pilgrims were sick and in need of nursing care. In 1217, thanks to the proceeds from salvaging a French ship after a local sea battle, the church you see today was built. It consists of a nave and a chancel (on the far side as you approach the building), with another chapel attached alongside the chancel. Surrounding the church were almshouses for local 'brothers' and 'sisters' (Hospitallians), who provided care for the sick pilgrims.

By 1773 the cottages were dilapidated and were rebuilt, with thatch replaced by tiles. The church was restored by George Gilbert Scott and his son in the 1880s (around the same time that St Bartholomew's chapel in Rochester was restored by his grandson, Giles). One of the 16

Kent Tour

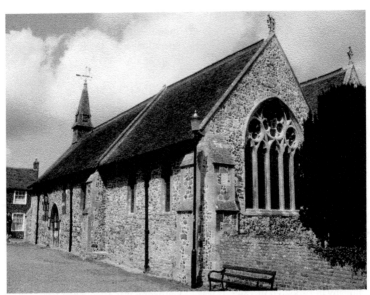

St Bartholomew's Hospital in Sandwich, built in 1217 to care for pilgrims on their way to Becket's tomb in Canterbury

almshouse residents is still selected to be Master of the hospital using a centuries-old system known as 'pricking the master': each trustee indicates their choice by pricking a list of Brothers using a bodkin. It is unclear how the hospital Matron is selected.

Return to your car and continue away from Sandwich. After 800 m turn left at the roundabout along Deal Road (A258). In four miles, when you enter Deal, follow signs to the town centre, where the second day of this tour ends.

Day Three: Deal to London

Highlights

- two cottage hospitals (Deal, Betteshanger)
- the third Royal Naval Hospital built in England (Deal)
- a fine Art Deco general hospital (Kent & Canterbury Hospital)
- 19th century workhouse infirmary (Canterbury)
- medieval hospitals for sick pilgrims (St John's, Eastbridge)
- remains of one of the largest cathedral infirmaries (Canterbury)
- medieval leper hospital (St Nicholas's Hospital, Harbledown)

The first site to visit is in the centre of Deal in Wellington Road, near the southern end of the pedestrianised High Street. No. 11 (Victoria Lodge), built in 1863, was the **Deal & Walmer Dispensary & Infirmary**. It was unusual in combining a dispensary (established four years earlier) and inpatient beds. Despite the name, it was a cottage hospital. As in Ramsgate, the five beds were primarily for injured seamen (who paid for their care), although others were admitted. The name was changed in 1897 for two reasons: Queen Victoria's diamond jubilee that year, and financial pressure that had led to the introduction of a provident (insurance) scheme for the dispensary in 1877. The result was one of the longest hospital names in England, Deal & Walmer Provident Dispensary and Infirmary and Victoria Hospital. The building was extended in 1904 by linking to an adjoining house to provide accommodation for nurses. Despite now having 10 beds and two cots, the demand for inpatient care could not be met, and in 1923 the hospital moved to new premises, which you will see soon.

Drive down Wellington Road, turn right into Victoria Road and then immediately left (Sondes Road). At the sea front, turn right, which takes you back to Victoria Road. Turn left, passing Deal Castle, and park after 50 m. The magnificent façade you see was the **Royal Naval Hospital**. It was the third such hospital to be built in England, constructed in 1795. Cross-wings were added as ward blocks in 1809, and two years later the central block was replaced with a design by Edward Holl that has a pediment and clock tower. It displays features that were advanced for their time, such as windows opposite each other to encourage ventilation.

Walk round to the rear and you can see the projecting blocks containing stairs, sanitary facilities and nurses' accommodation. Separate from the main building were staff residences, a mortuary and a block for the insane. In 1930 the hospital closed as part of a nationwide reorganisation of Royal Naval hospitals. The building became the home of the Royal Marines' School of Music, which remained until 1996. It is now private residences.

Kent Tour

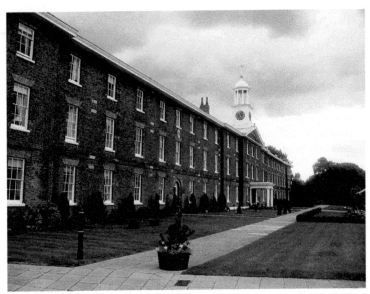

The magnificent central block of the Royal Naval Hospital in Deal, built in 1811 facing the North Sea

Return to your car and continue south for about 800 m before turning right into Cornwall Road. After going under the railway, it becomes Hamilton Road. Turn right into Mill Road and take the third on the left, Allenby Avenue. At the end you will see the **Deal, Walmer & District Victoria War Memorial Hospital** across the junction. Drive into the car park and stop. The new name recognised the 600 local men killed in World War I. The two-storey building is much more modest than that of Margate & District Hospital (built seven years later). However, it had its own radiology department, and in the 1930s local support led to the addition of a nurses' home, more wards and a minor operating theatre. Unlike in Margate, it remained a cottage hospital. During its first year

in the NHS in 1948, Claire Rayner embarked on her illustrious career here as a cadet nurse. The hospital underwent significant expansion and improvements in 1985 and continues to function as a 36-bedded cottage hospital with a minor injuries clinic and specialist clinics.

Leave the hospital grounds and turn right onto London Road (A258, Sandwich). After 2.2 miles turn left (Betteshanger). After one mile turn right to Eastry. (Ignore the road that then goes off to the left to Betteshanger.) After 1.3 miles turn left onto the A256, and at the roundabout take the exit to Eastry. After about 500 m, at the bottom of the hill, turn left and park. The small flintstone building back on the other side of the main road (Crossways Cottage) was

Cottage hospitals

The first cottage hospital was established in Cranleigh, Surrey in 1859, and over the next 70 years 600 were developed in small towns throughout England. Their key feature was that local GPs could admit and care for patients. Avoiding admission to city hospitals meant that patients benefited from staying near their homes while GPs gained in status and kept the fees that would otherwise have gone to city doctors.

Usually, one GP acted as the medical superintendent, either permanently or in rotation. On average, there were 15 beds, although the number varied. Pregnancy, lunacy and infectious cases were initially excluded, although surgical operations were often performed. Funding came from several sources: legacies or donations from philanthropists; local subscribers (similar to voluntary hospitals); working-class weekly subscriptions; and, unlike city hospitals, patient co-payments.

The aim was that cottage hospitals should resemble a poor man's cottage, based on a romantic view of a 19th century home. Their construction coincided with the development of the Arts & Crafts movement, noted for vernacular styles and building methods that reflected the local style. Typically, the ground floor would contain a kitchen, sitting-room and scullery, while the first floor had four to six well-ventilated rooms. Some commemorated famous people, others were established to commemorate Queen Victoria's golden jubilee in 1897, and others were memorials to soldiers killed in World War I.

In the 20th century, they increased in size and some introduced specialist care overseen by doctors from nearby city hospitals. Maternity care was introduced widely from 1918, providing a local alternative to maternity homes. During the inter-war years, they faced growing criticism about their quality compared with city hospitals. While many have closed in recent decades, some survive, and some have been enhanced to become general hospitals.

built as the **Betteshanger Cottage Hospital**. Walk back along the main road to see the front of this quintessential cottage hospital. It was built in 1873, designed by George Devey, whose Old English country house style inspired the later creation of the Arts & Crafts Movement. It consisted of a central entrance and two small wards, each with seven beds. Unfortunately, a rather unsympathetic replacement of the leaded, mullion windows and enlargement of the basement windows have detracted from its original appearance. The hospital survived only until 1897, when it became a nursing home. It served as an Auxiliary War Hospital during World War I.

Turn round and continue up the hill into Eastry. At the top, take the first left into Mill Lane and park just after the Fire Station. In 2012

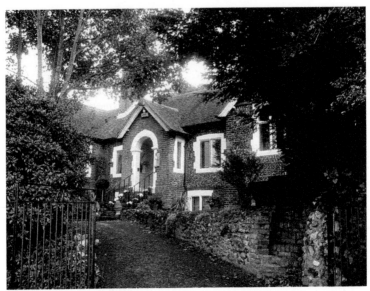

Betteshanger Cottage Hospital (in Eastry), designed by George Devey in 1873, whose work inspired the Arts & Crafts Movement, and now a private home

the buildings on the left side of the road were awaiting redevelopment. The first red-brick building was the original **Eastry Parish Workhouse**. Next to it is a larger brick building with a grand façade. Beyond that is the old workhouse chapel, designed by George Devey in 1873 in the Early English style and complete with a double bell-cote. You can get a better view if you walk up the driveway just beyond the chapel.

Little remains of the large workhouse built in 1835 for the newly formed Eastry Poor Law Union. You can see the arched entrance, to the right of the church, which led into a large quadrangle of two-storey buildings, of which only the north side survives. Designed by William Spanton, it could

accommodate 500 destitute people. The workhouse was extended first in 1871 with the addition of a large infirmary containing 104 beds, and again in 1901 with three small isolation wards for fevers, TB and smallpox.

In 1930 responsibility for the workhouse infirmary transferred to Kent County Council. It was renamed Eastry Hospital in 1942 when it became a facility for those with learning difficulties, a role it continued to fulfil within the NHS until 1985. Having been left abandoned for 20 years, most of the hospital was demolished in 2008. Two small intermediate care facilities have been constructed to the west, thus continuing the tradition of health care on this site.

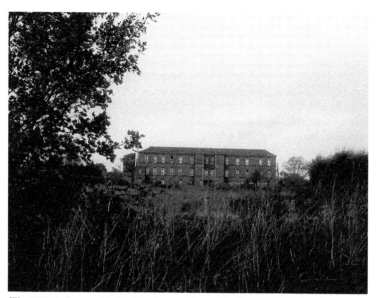

The 1871 infirmary block of the former Eastry Workhouse, which dominated the landscape until its demolition in 2008

Turn and drive back to the main road. Turn left and drive on through Eastry. After passing the Village Hall on the left, take the left fork (Woodnesborough Lane) to the left of the Post Office, to Staple. After one mile turn right at a T-junction and immediately left to Staple, three miles away. At Staple continue another two miles to Wingham, where you join the A257 to Canterbury (about six miles).

On the outskirts of Canterbury, look out for St Martin's Hospital on the left. Turn into the second entrance, and after 50 m stop, overlooking the main hospital entrance. In 1899 Canterbury Borough Council purchased Stone House, complete with 55 acres, here outside the city to meet the requirements of the 1890 Lunacy

Act, which made local councils responsible for providing asylums. The collection of two-storey, red-brick buildings you can see were built to create the **Canterbury Borough Asylum**. To see more, take the left fork uphill towards Dudley Venables, turn right at the T-junction, take the second on the right and stop after 30m. During the early decades of the 20th century, several additional ward blocks were constructed, such as Gregory House to your right and beyond that another grand block. In 1948 the asylum passed to the NHS and, like so many others, was renamed (St Martin's Hospital) to reduce any stigma associated with being a patient here. It continues to provide mental health services.

Turn round and follow the 'Way Out' signs to return to the A257. Turn

Kent Tour

left and descend into Canterbury. After the road flattens out, note the row of almshouses on the left, opposite the prison, built in 1657. About 300 m further on, you reach a roundabout. To the right was the site of the Kent & Canterbury Hospital from 1793 to 1937. In an act of vandalism, the imposing 18th century building was demolished in 1971.

Take the first exit from the roundabout, and at the traffic lights carry straight on. After 200 m, at the next set of traffic lights, go straight over into Nunnery Fields and take the fourth right, George Roche Road. Turn left immediately into a new housing development and park. Walk along the road in front of the long building that was on the right as you drove in. This was the front of the **Canterbury Workhouse**,

designed by Hezekiah Marshall and built in 1848–50. It formed one side of a quadrangle accommodating 400 inmates. Walk to the end to see the beautifully restored 70-bed infirmary, added in 1883.

Retrace your steps and go round to the back of the workhouse quadrangle. The back has been replaced with new buildings, but a gap in the middle allows you to see a single-storey building (which was the dining room) projecting from the front block and dividing the quadrangle into two courtyards, enabling the two sexes to be segregated. On inclusion into the NHS in 1948, it became Nunnery Fields Hospital and provided care for the elderly until 2001.

On leaving the site, turn right into George Roche Road and then

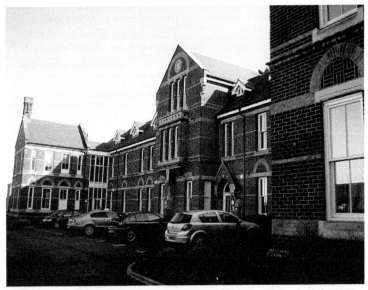

The former Canterbury Workhouse Infirmary at Nunnery Fields, built in 1883 and now sensitively converted to housing

right along South Canterbury Road. At the end, turn left (Ethelbert Road), and after about 100 m turn right through the original Art Deco entrance to the **Kent & Canterbury Hospital**. Drive along the avenue of horse chestnut trees to the fine 1937 hospital building. This is one of the finest Art Deco hospital buildings in the country, a period marked by few new buildings, reflecting the dire financial state of most voluntary general hospitals. The design is unusual in being a triangle with a block projecting from each corner. The clock tower emerges from the centre of the triangle. Some of the symmetry of the building was lost when the main entrance was moved from its central position, where it had been surmounted by a modified Maltese cross. The separate four-storey buildings to the left with a striking chequer-board façade were staff residences. Over the past 70 years, the buildings that have been added on this site have paid no regard to the simple, pure lines of the original hospital.

Drive back to the road, turn right and then left at the T-junction. After 200 m, when you reach a roundabout, turn right along the ring road. Go straight on at the next roundabout and take the first exit at the second (Chaucer) roundabout into Tourtel Road. At the next roundabout, turn left into Northgate and park in the car park on the right.

Walk to the right along Northgate. About 200 m on the right is the entrance to **St John's Hospital**,

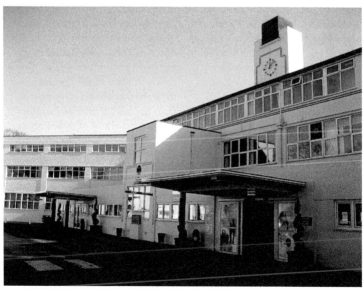

One of the few Art Deco hospitals, Kent and Canterbury Hospital was built in 1937. The original central entrance was replaced with two lateral entrances

now a collection of almshouses. This medieval hospital was founded by Archbishop Lanfranc in 1085 for aged, sick and poor Saxons, and it could accommodate 100 patients who were cared for by 'watchers'. Their spiritual needs were met by chaplains from St Gregory's Priory across the road. Due to fire in the 14th century, only some ruins remain of the original hospital. And all that remains of the late-15th century replacement is the gatehouse. The almshouses, which can be glimpsed through the gates, were replaced in the 19th century.

Continue along Northgate, and after 300 m follow the road round to the right. Take King Street (to the right of the leaning building), which curves to the left and becomes Best Lane before ending on the High Street. To the right is the beautiful, medieval flint-stone building of **Eastbridge Hospital** (open Mon–Sat 10.00–17.00 h). It was founded in 1190, about 20 years after the murder of Thomas Becket, to meet the needs of the growing number of sick pilgrims visiting his shrine in the belief that it had healing powers. It takes its name from the neighbouring bridge, for which it was responsible (until the 18th century) and from which it gained income from those using it. The low entrance resulted from the need to raise the road. The undercroft served as an infirmary containing 12 beds. A small chantry chapel was built at right angles to the infirmary, to which, unlike in most medieval hospitals, there was no easy access. The women who nursed the sick

pilgrims had to be over 40 years of age. Extraordinarily for the time, pregnant women were, from 1342, allowed to stay. It changed function to an almshouse in the 16th century.

When you leave, turn right and then third left (Mercery Lane), which takes you to the main entrance (Christ Church Gate) to **Canterbury Cathedral** (open Mon–Sat 9.00–17.00 h; Sun 12.30–14.30 h). The first cathedral established here by Augustine in 597 was destroyed by fire in 1067. Three years later, Lanfranc (an Italian) was appointed archbishop and set about building a new cathedral and monastery, which opened in 1077. Following another fire in 1174, the Gothic building you see today was constructed.

To the north-east of the main building, the infirmary was constructed. Having entered the grounds, walk anti-clockwise round to the east end of the cathedral. As you pass the apse, you will see five massive ruined arches that seem to be striding out across the lawns from the main buildings. Together with a parallel row of arches, these supported the roof of the infirmary hall. The infirmary was actually even longer, as there were originally seven arches. And as you can see, the building did not end there. Beyond are the arches of the infirmary chapel. The sick were seeking, and the monks were providing, spiritual as much as physical salvation. Given that many patients would have been seriously ill, preparation for the 'next life' and minimising time spent in purgatory would have been

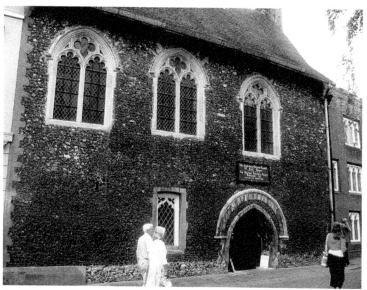

Eastbridge Hospital, founded in 1190 to provide care for sick pilgrims visiting Becket's shrine. Raising the road level has reduced the height of the doorway

uppermost in their minds. Demand on beds in the infirmary would have increased considerably as belief in the healing powers of Becket's shrine developed after 1170.

At the far end of the infirmary hall is a doorway that takes you into the infirmary cloisters. On the far side is a passageway (locutorium) that connects to the main cathedral cloisters and through to the west front of the cathedral.

On leaving the Cathedral, turn right along Sun Street (which becomes Palace Street) to return to your car. Turn left out of the car park and then right at the roundabout. At the next roundabout, turn right (second exit) and stay on the ring road until you reach the fourth roundabout, where you should take the first exit (towards the A2). After 800 m take the exit to Harbledown. As the road descends into the village, you will see **St Nicholas's Hospital** on the left. Park and walk up the path to the church.

When 'the leper hospital' was founded by Archbishop Lanfranc in 1085, Harbledown was just a clearing in the Forest of Blean on the London to Dover road. The site was chosen as it was well outside Canterbury and its spring water was believed to have medicinal properties. You enter the churchyard through the 14th century gatehouse, built to accommodate clerics. The beautiful church was surrounded by wattle huts that housed as many as 100 people with leprosy. With the disappearance of the disease in the 14th century, the

Kent Tour

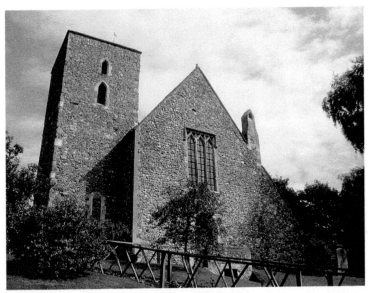

St Nicholas's Hospital for lepers was founded in 1085 at Harbledown, well outside the Canterbury city walls

establishment was converted into almshouses. The present houses were built in 1840 and accommodate 16 residents and one nurse.

Parts of the church (the west entrance, tower and the nave) are Norman, with the north aisle added in the 12th century. If you can see inside (by prior appointment), there are two interesting features: the floor slopes from east to west to facilitate cleaning and disinfection after services; and until the 19th century, there was a screen running the length of the nave separating the sexes. Henry II's pledge to donate 8 ounces of gold or silver annually (part of his repentance for the murder of Becket) was still being honoured in 1977, although the gift went to the Kent & Canterbury Hospital.

Return to your car and continue on through Harbledown. After 400 m you can join the A2050, which takes you to the A2 (London). After five miles the A2 joins the M2 to London to complete your tour.

Index

Note: page numbers in **bold** refer to information contained in boxes, pages numbers in *italics* refer to photographs and illustrations.